Trust me, I'm a health manager

Greg Sheridan + Charlotte Rastan + Dan Foulkes

www.institute.nhs.uk

A catalogue record for this book is available from the British Library

ISBN 978-1-906535-72-8

Design by The Team

Printed and bound in Great Britain by Bookmarque

PEFC
PEFC/16-33-281

For everyone

"Good managers are absolutely vital to the NHS. High quality dignified patient care goes hand in hand with excellent leadership and that's demonstrated on a daily basis in every part of the NHS."

Doctor Peter Carter
Chief Executive and General Secretary of the Royal College of Nursing

"Perhaps like any organisation, the NHS has its different camps. Poor relationships between managers and clinicians make for a great soap opera, and there are places where they still exist. But things are changing. When we learn about best practice, often it's emerging from these two camps working side by side. And more and more managers are beginning their careers as clinicians. It's time we recognised and properly championed the critical role this partnership can play in improving services."

Professor Bernard Crump
Chief Executive, NHS Institute for Innovation and Improvement

"A world-class NHS needs world-class doctors and managers. Thankfully, we have both and we know that when clinicians and managers work well together we can provide the very best healthcare for our patients. Doctors are becoming increasingly involved in NHS management, either as managers or through working closely with management colleagues, leading to a better understanding by all concerned of the pressures facing all members of the health team. The Royal College of Physicians believes medical leadership is vital in driving up the quality of care for patients."

Professor Ian Gilmore
President of the Royal College of Physicians

"To make the NHS work for patients and the public, clinicians and managers must work together as one. They must share a set of values, a vision and a determination to ensure that finite NHS resources – the public's money – is used most effectively to create the best quality services possible, most closely aligned to patients' needs. This means that doctors must gain high-level skills of management and leadership alongside their clinical work – not as an optional extra – but as a matter of course."

Professor Jenny Simpson OBE
Chief Executive, British Association of Medical Managers

Preface

THINGS HAPPEN WHEN you're least expecting them. One minute the NHS doesn't really cross your mind, then suddenly it's everywhere. We all know of somebody who's experienced the wonders of the National Health Service at some time in their life: a brother gets taken to A&E to remove the toy lorry tyre he's somehow managed to wedge up his nose, a friend breaks a leg during football and a neighbour has his appendix removed. Then, of course, there's the really serious stuff, too. But it's rare when you're writing a book that everyone around you seems strangely connected to what you're writing. During the months it's taken to plan, structure, research and compose this book, one of our parents suffered a broken femur, while another was diagnosed with Parkinsonism; one friend caught Meningitis, luckily just the viral strain, and another gave birth to bouncing twins, Vincent and Laila. The NHS touches all of us.

The thing about the NHS is it's just there, lurking quietly in the background, yet ready to spring into action the moment it's called upon. But until it does, we tend to forget about it, take it for granted.

And that, perhaps, is the greatest accolade you could ever give to any business or organisation. You trust it so much and know that it is always going to be there when you need it, that you don't have to spend time wondering about it. Just like that ultra-reliable car sitting outside that starts first time, every time, come rain, snow or heatwave.

This whole project has actually been about good management. Not just in terms of the subject matter, but also in the way it's been carried out. Without it, it simply wouldn't, couldn't, have happened. A challenging, immovable deadline; uncovering great stories and tracking down contributors for interviews; carrying out background research; and then actually writing the book.

But it was also great management on the part of Peter Mills and Lyndal Kearney at The Team, and Nicola Fair and Angela Antolini at the NHS Institute for Innovation and Improvement, who co-ordinated and project managed the whole thing. They knew when to email and when to leave well alone. It's called trust. With it you can move mountains. Without it, things just don't happen. Even when things didn't quite go according to plan – when do they ever? – there were no frantic, ranting phone calls, just a friendly voice offering advice and support as to how we could work together to make the best of it. Thanks also go to designer David Recchia at The Team and to Dave Thornton who led the Building Leadership Capacity team.

Finally, our thanks go to all the contributors, without whom this book would be little more than a series of blank and uninspiring pages. So, to Steve Allder, Chris Edwards, Debbie Taylor, James Hobbs, Salma Yasmeen, Antony Sumara, Carol Farrow, Sarah Chalmers, Mark Johnston, Valerie James, Neda Hormozi, Stephen Langford, Barbara Stocking, Olivia Amartey, Roshelle Ramkisson, Dave Sherwood and Wayne Elliott, thank you for your insights, thoughts, stories and time.

Greg Sheridan + Charlotte Rastan + Dan Foulkes

About the authors

DAN FOULKES and **GREG SHERIDAN** were originally journalists writing in national broadsheets and for magazines on marketing and branding, and were also the editors of leading professional trade publications on advertising and design. They formed a writing partnership in 1999 and became Milknosugar, and have created communications for dozens of high profile clients including the Royal Opera House, Jaguar and the Virgin Group. Both have family members who work, or have worked, in the NHS in clinical roles.

CHARLOTTE RASTAN trained as a cub reporter with a London newspaper group before going freelance to write features for the broadsheets and magazines. She now works as a copywriter and journalist for a wide range of clients in the public and private sectors.

Contents

A dream come true

"**TAKE PRIDE IN** the fact that, despite our financial and economic anxieties, we are still able to do the most civilised thing in the world: put the welfare of the sick in front of every other consideration."

Those inspirational words were spoken by Nye Bevan, Secretary for Health, on 9th February 1948. Five months later, on 5th July, the remarkable dream of a National Health Service, the Western world's first free health system for an entire population, was a reality. It was a momentous day of celebration, optimism, hope, and the start of the greatest and most beneficial political achievement this country will probably ever witness. If you can't see where you came from it's hard to see where you're going. The route of NHS management across the years is a compass for where we are and where we will go.

The chain of life

CHRIS EDWARDS IS a policeman in his thirties, based in Liverpool, living on the Wirral. Normal guy. Normal life. But his world was shattered when he rode into a new reality.

"1st July 2003. A date I'll never forget. 6.40 in the morning, riding my first motorbike, a little 125. The weather was drizzly and the road conditions were damp. I was travelling to our police HQ at the port. As I pulled away from a set of traffic lights there was a bend. Out of the corner of my eye I saw a car travelling at about 50mph in a 30mph zone. He lost control, spun and smashed right into me.

"Time slowed down. The last thing I remember before the impact was that this car was in my way, and I wasn't going to miss it. I thought that was it. As a police officer I've been to accidents like this, and people don't walk away from them. I went over the top of the bike and was flung 20 to 30 feet down the road. As I lay on the tarmac I found I had problems breathing because of my anti-fogging mask under my helmet, and as I looked at my right arm I saw it was all bent out of shape. I could feel pins and needles in my legs, but I couldn't actually feel my legs. I was in shock.

"I heard a car stop behind me and a guy came up and said: 'Don't worry I'm a policeman. You're going to be fine. Don't move.' Then I heard a woman's voice saying the same thing. There was a paramedic, too, with full kit, from the Mersey River Rescue. I was losing quite a lot of blood. She tried to keep an open airway and to stem the blood loss. They found out I was a policeman with the port police so they came out in numbers as well.

"I could hear the sirens coming when the ambulance arrived. They put my legs and arms in splints, giving me gas and air to help with the pain. They put a neck collar on me and loaded me into the back of the ambulance. When they moved me I was in more pain than I've ever experienced. It was unbearable, but I didn't lose consciousness.

"I was taken to the Royal Liverpool hospital. I remember the journey there; all the equipment rattling and siren screaming. There was a paramedic in the back of the ambulance with me who checked my heart and breathing and tried to keep control of the blood loss.

"I remember arriving at the hospital, being wheeled to the door and thinking: 'I've got this far and I'm still alive.' They have a specialised trauma team for poly trauma cases like mine, who they can call in from all areas of the hospital. They were waiting: orthopaedic surgeons, physiotherapists, trauma nurses. One of the surgeons had passed by the accident scene on his way to work.

"My colleagues informed my fiancée, Ruth, and collected her from home. She came to the hospital and we talked for a bit while I was in casualty. They put me through x-rays first and a full body scan. They had problems getting me through the CT scanner because my body had swelled up so much. I felt like Mr Blobby. I thought: 'This is not me.'"

In the space of a matter of hours Chris Edwards' life had been transformed. He was under the care of two orthopaedic consultants: Mr Badri Narayan and Mr Durai Nayagam. Whether he would survive and in what condition he'd emerge from the operating room was now down to the surgical team.

"They took me down to theatre where I remained for 13 hours. The surgery was done by four teams of surgeons. My injuries were extensive: right open forearm fracture, in two places; fractured open right femur; open right tibia and fibula; fractured wrist, left hand; and fractured left femur and knee cap. Apart from a cut caused by my crash helmet on my chin, my neck and spinal column were perfect.

"But my limbs were mangled, so there were multiple procedures. The first, on my left arm, was to clean the wound, remove the bone that had road grit in and put a plate on that. On my right femur, I had lost a lot of bone from road grit and contamination, so they had to insert a long nail from top to bottom. My lower right leg had to be cleaned and any contaminated bone removed. Another nail was put in my left femur and my left wrist was wired together.

"I was suffering from something called 'Compartment Syndrome' on my lower right leg, so they sliced away lots of muscle because the blood pressure inside was building up so much I would have lost my leg if it had not been released. I had an external fixator frame fitted, with four huge bolts going through my leg and a bar on top to stabilise it. I was pumped full of antibiotics and put into a drug-induced coma for three days."

On 4th July, Independence Day, Chris Edwards opened his eyes. "When I was in the coma one of the physios came up, examined me and ordered a wheelchair there and then. That's good long-term planning. I woke up in ICU to find out I was bandaged from head to toe. And I had patient-administered morphine to keep on top of the pain.

"I was in intensive care for a further week and had another op; a skin graft. At the end, I had lost a significant amount of blood, bone, muscle and skin. But everything was explained to me. The two surgeons who were in charge were the nicest, most gentle people

I have ever met. If I could give out knighthoods, they would both get one. They were really pleased with the way the surgery had gone, and were amazed that I had come through it as well as I had.

"There was a rota of intensive care nurses, one-to-one care night and day. They brought in a specialist plastic surgeon to look at the skin grafts. I think he came from a London hospital because he brought his own equipment. He just looked at me and said: 'Let's get it done.'"

The surgery was an outstanding success and Chris was transferred to the High Dependency Unit. Then onto the orthopaedic reception ward, and finally to the ortho recovery ward where he stayed for four months. Throughout this time, Chris was receiving 12 units of blood; roughly all the blood in the human body.

He explains: "On the ortho ward, the nurses are all specialists. I was told I had lost 10 centimetres of bone from my left leg. They started physio on me straight away to keep my joints flexible. They brought in a special air-filled bed that moves you so you don't get bed sores. They told me it costs £60,000. I'm 6'4", too tall for the bed, so they went out and got this specialist engineer to fit an extension for me. The bed was all electronic so I could sit myself up or lay myself down. The bed would even turn me over. They also brought in a machine to exercise my knee so it didn't seize up.

"They said they would have to wait a month or so for the skin grafts to settle. Then they started getting me out of bed and sitting me up in a chair. It was exhausting and painful. I had to go for more surgery for my left wrist because the wire wasn't taking properly. My legs had no strength to support me, but Mr Nayagam said if I behaved myself there was every possibility I could go back to work. I've got to say that what really got me through all this were the times my family and friends came in. Ruth was a pillar of strength throughout. She went through hell and back. I owe her everything really.

"I was going down to occupational therapy once a day to build up the strength in my arms and learning how to use special crutches that take the weight off your forearms. They had this 'torture machine' which they could set up to simulate different tasks like pouring tea or taking a lid off a jar. Unfortunately, one of the fractures in my right arm wasn't healing and I managed to bend one of the plates in my arm, so I had to have a bone graft from my pelvis and place it in the arm to promote healing. They used two plastic foam moulds on my hand, one to keep it open at night and one for normal day time use.

"At this time I also had my external fixator removed and an Ilizarov external fixator frame fitted to my lower right leg. It was explained to me that this device would be used to re-grow the bone I had lost in the accident by 1mm a day. This would be done by adjusting four bolts, four times a day with a spanner."

With massive personal effort and the support of his fiancée, friends, family and care team, the day dawned when Chris could finally go home. "When they discharged me, I could get up and down stairs on my bottom. I was getting quite good at it. They sent the physio and the occupational therapist round to my home to see what equipment I needed."

Recovering from such a severe trauma, physically and psychologically, is never an easy path, however, as Chris discovered. "I became an outpatient at the end of October. My future mother-in-law took a load of my trousers, split the seams and attached Velcro so I could get dressed with the frame on.

"Just before Christmas I came down with a severe bout of depression. I was very upset and very angry. I was prescribed anti-depressants to help stabilise my moods, which I was on for 12 months. Normally in our day-to-day lives we do things that give us pleasure. But if you sit at home all day with nothing to do, you are not getting any of that positive feedback. They told me that that was why I was depressed."

The aftercare continued as Chris recovered. "Twice a week an ambulance came to pick me up and take me to the Royal. The physio department was excellent. It was led by a gentleman called Giles. He and his team knew everything about the Ilizarov frame. A large advantage I found with these physio sessions was the opportunity I had to talk to other patients who had been going through the same experience I was going though. A number of times I was asked by Mr Narayan and Mr Nayagam to go up and talk to patients who were about to have this frame put on and tell them about the practicalities of it.

"The district nurse team came to me every 10 days to clean the pins through the leg. Since there is a large risk of infection through the pin sites, it was a two-hour procedure to change the gauze and bandages. On top of that I was part of an experiment using ultra sonic waves to increase the maturity of the bone. I was told to put as much weight through the leg as possible. They were trying all sorts of research on me, but I didn't mind. After all, that's how medical advances are made."

In January 2005, 19 months after the accident, Chris returned to work, and in August married Ruth. Around that time he also met, and shook hands with, the man who changed the course of his life on that drizzly morning on 1st July 2003. He was charged and convicted with dangerous driving.

Chris' mobility is now about 90–95%. "I've since trained as a counter-terrorist search officer. There's nothing I can't do. I climb up lorries and gangways to ships. My job is with the Port of Liverpool Police. We deal with all types of crime including assaults, theft and a lot of searches on ships, HGVs and buildings. I work closely with Customs & Excise and other agencies.

"The whole thing has made me more philosophical about life. I think of it as a real learning experience. There were an awful lot of dedicated people involved in putting me back together. I was surprised at the organisational skills that were behind it. If I needed something, it was there, from the equipment to the ambulance. Everyone was fantastic, but I really would like to thank the sister in charge of the ward, a nurse called Sue Moffat, who sang all the time, my physio team, and, of course, the two consultants. At my last appointment before I was discharged I thanked them for giving me back my life.

"I've got to say, the teamwork was excellent. They went way beyond their job remit, looking after my wellbeing as well as my physical care. If there was something wrong with the frame, one of the Mr Ns would come down and sort it out. And when I came down with an infection, one of the consultants came in on a Sunday. The team told him and he came straight in. That was the sort of person he was.

"I do get ribbed all the time at work. Because I've got so much metal in me, they're always threatening to throw me into the scrap metal pile as they would receive a fair price for the metal still in me! And every time I'm near a magnet they tell me not to get too close."

Paramedic. Ambulance. Specialised trauma team. Orthopaedic surgeons. Physiotherapists. Trauma nurses. X-rays. Full body scan. Ilizarov external fixator frame. Antibiotics. Wheelchair. Patient-administered morphine. Intensive care nurses. Specialist plastic surgeon. Special air-filled bed. Specialist engineer. Occupational therapy. Crutches. Anti-depressants. District nurse team.

These were the links in Chris Edwards' journey back to life. But the chain is built by NHS managers, co-ordinating and overseeing every aspect of a patient's path, bringing it all together and making it happen. They are the missing link. Rarely seen. Always there.

Another chain of events

CHRIS EDWARDS IS a policeman in his thirties, based in Liverpool, living on the Wirral. Normal guy. Normal life. But his world was shattered when he rode into a new reality. A reality without NHS managers. No link in the chain. Just imagine...

1st July 2003. The ambulance arrived late and without the necessary equipment. The specialised trauma team was missing key members. The air-filled bed was still on order. There were no spare wheelchairs and all the district nurses were on holiday at the same time. No one had co-ordinated the theatre lists to allow four surgeons to be available to operate on him.

60 years of NHS managers

1948 At the birth of the NHS, there are two hospital management systems: those run by local authorities and those run as voluntary hospitals. They have to come together under one new management structure – the hospital management committee.

The people in the top jobs are called group secretaries, with hospital secretaries being the next step down. The role of hospital secretaries is very wide ranging: running the whole hospital in partnership with nursing and medical colleagues.

The most junior managers are clerks and their duties could include weighing out slabs of Genoa cake for patients.

1948–1974 For 26 years, there is no national reorganisation of the NHS, and structures remain remarkably unchanged. The first management trainees join the National Administrative Training Scheme in 1956.

1974 A new structure is put in place throughout the NHS, creating four layers of management: hospitals, districts, areas and regions.

The title of secretary is dropped in favour of administrator. The district administrator becomes the chief executive of the district health authority, with a much wider range of health services, including child and public health.

One of the underlying principles of the change is to align health authorities and local government, promoting – in modern-day jargon – joined-up thinking.

Power moves away from hospital managers to the regions, prompting Labour Health Secretary Richard Crossman to complain that regional health authorities are like "semi-autonomous governors in the Persian empire – they do what they damn well like".

1979 The conservative government, led by Margaret Thatcher, aims to boost the power of health managers.

1982 It abolishes the area health authorities.

1983 A turning point comes when businessman Sir Roy Griffiths, working with a team of three advisers, reports on management within the NHS. He recommends strong management throughout the NHS. His recommendations are adopted wholesale the following year, leading to the creation for the first time of general managers throughout the health service.

Griffiths spells the end of consensus management. Managers become involved in strategic and system management. They are professional and autonomous, with clear lines of accountability – the chief executive carries the can.

One of the medical journals of the time criticises the Griffiths revolution, saying that giving power to administrators was like giving whisky to Red Indians.

1990s Health Secretary Kenneth Clarke begins to hold the NHS to account for spending and for waiting lists, through a new mechanism: the internal market.

Purchasers are able to hold providers to account. Newly created hospital trusts reintroduce the hospital board, with non-executive directors drawn from a wide range of backgrounds. Each trust also has a medical director and a nursing director on the board. Chief executives have to carry their boards, including these knowledgeable and expert clinical and nursing leads, with them.

Targets provoke strong disagreement, as managers are accused of interfering with clinical matters. This coincides with a period of industrial unrest: nurses protest about low wages and cleaners about contracting out services.

1997 Tony Blair wins the general election and his government pledges to get rid of the internal market and inject cash into the NHS.

2001 A report into the management of paediatric cardiac care at Bristol Royal Infirmary revolutionises clinical governance. In future, there are to be no 'no go' areas for managers.

A new code of conduct is introduced for managers to underline their accountability. They can lose their jobs for failing to meet targets.

2008 At the 60th anniversary of the founding of the NHS, foundation trusts and the commissioner's role in primary care trusts are among the hot management topics of the day.

Living the dream

IN THE 21ST CENTURY it's all too easy to take for granted the presence of the NHS in so many different aspects of our lives, but as an organisational structure it is truly extraordinary. Its shape changes constantly, but the driving imperative to provide the best healthcare possible remains the same. The NHS has always been about passing on the baton in a relay of care to look after every man, woman and child in the country, each and every day. Managing it, to ensure that the vision remains robust is an awesome responsibility and an incredible challenge due to the unimaginable size and complexity of the NHS in 2008 and beyond, compared to the organisation that was born in 1948. The people who choose to be part of this process should be proud to take on such an admirable, demanding and, on occasion, thankless task. Without them, where would our country be? After all, the NHS is a matter of life and death.

Nothing physically changed the day after the NHS was launched. No new hospitals sprang up out of the blue, and there was no sudden influx of new doctors, nurses, hospital beds or equipment. Yet socially and emotionally, everything changed. For the first time, everyone had exactly the same right to free health and medicine. All NHS staff were salaried; doctors, dentists, opticians and pharmacists remained self-employed; and community-based services such as midwifery, health visits and welfare clinics, were unified and united. One for all, and all for one. For the first time hospitals, doctors, nurses, pharmacists, dentists and opticians were brought together under the auspices of a single organisation where their skills, training and opinions were available, free of charge, to everyone in Britain; even to people visiting the country.

Recognition of the crucial role of structures and management in empowering the NHS first arose during the 1960s. Treatment improved with the creation of better drugs. Polio vaccine became available. Dialysis for renal failure and chemotherapy for certain cancers were developed. The problem was, as with most medical advances, this all added to costs. GP practices became better housed and better staffed, and doctors formed partnerships and groups, resulting in the development of the modern group practice.

With the increasing complexity of the structures and challenges within the NHS, management began to assume a more prominent role to become a focus for improvement. Consequently, the Cogwheel Report of 1967 sought to encourage the involvement of clinicians in management. Hospital Activity Analysis was introduced to provide better patient-based information, and medical staff were grouped by speciality to explore clinical and managerial issues. The Salmon Report of 1967 built on this with recommendations for developing the senior nursing staff structure and raising its profile within hospital management.

From the end of the 1960s and into the 1970s, medical progress continued with advances including the widening application of endoscopy and the development of CAT scanning. Transplant surgery and genetic engineering were both beginning to revolutionise medical possibilities and thinking. ICUs and kidney dialysis became widely available. In general practice, the GPs' charter encouraged the formation of primary healthcare teams, new group practice premises and an increase in the number of health centres. New hospitals sprang up nationwide with a massive positive impact on local health provision. Management and accountability tools took great strides forward with advances in information technology, leading to increasing computerisation and clinical budgeting.

This explosion in the provision of services meant that the NHS was experiencing change at an unprecedented level. However, it wasn't a fully balanced organisation as the distribution of its resources remained uneven. The solution lay in the establishment of the Resource Allocation Working Party in 1976, which devised a new system of allocation targets based on population, mortality and other factors. The NHS was evolving into an ever-more co-ordinated organisation to respond, at all levels, to the needs of an increasing population.

The focus coming out of the 1970s was the recognition of the financial constraints that the NHS had to operate under and making the most of its budgets in the face of new and complex technologies, which had encouraged rising expectations of the health service among an ageing population. The NHS' financial concerns were exacerbated by the oil crisis of 1978. This underlined the critical need for improvements in efficiency and management.

In 1983, Sir Roy Griffiths, then the managing director of Sainsbury's, was asked to "take a look" at manpower in the NHS. He explains: "I said it didn't make sense to look at the manpower. Quite clearly, if the manpower is out of control, you have got management problems." As a consequence his task became, instead, to "look at the management of the health service". He concluded that the NHS was institutionally stagnant, but that change and improvement was difficult to achieve within the existing structures. His recommendation was that a general management structure should be implemented throughout the NHS. The new structure was to be led by a supervisory board, chaired by the secretary for health, with a chief executive set below it to carry out its objectives and decisions and provide leadership to the organisation as a whole.

The Griffiths Report also challenged the notion that the NHS cannot be viewed like a business because it has no profit motive and should, therefore, be judged by wider social standards, which cannot be measured. It concluded: "These differences can be greatly over-stated. The clear similarities between NHS management and business management are much more important. In many organisations in the private sector, profit does not immediately impinge on large numbers of managers below board level. They are concerned with levels of service, quality of product, meeting budgets, cost improvement, productivity, motivating and rewarding staff, research and development, and the long-term viability of the undertaking."

The Griffiths Report led to the creation of general managers at all levels in the operation of the NHS from 1984 and the practice of recruiting widely from industries beyond the organisation to strengthen and enrich management. General (as opposed to consensus) management was introduced, and it aimed to erect three distinct pillars of governance: to provide one individual at every level of the organisation to be responsible, and to have authority and accountability, for planning and implementing decisions; to enable more flexibility in team structures; to encourage a greater emphasis on clear leadership. These were the roots of modern management structures and techniques within the NHS. As the then Secretary of State for Health and Social Services, Norman Fowler, commented: "The NHS is the largest undertaking in Western Europe. The service needs and deserves the very best management we can give it." The Griffiths reforms were not introduced without controversy and, in many ways and in many quarters, the debate about how best to manage the NHS continues today.

The monumental challenges that the NHS has faced since its conception don't go away: how to organise and fund it, where to direct resources to best effect, and how to balance the needs and expectations of patients, staff and taxpayers. Engaging with these challenges is what successive governments and management have done, and will always continue to have to do. The NHS is not perfect, but it does an outstanding job in countless ways. Nye Bevan put it simply: "We shall never have all we need. Expectations will always exceed capacity. The service must always be changing, growing and improving – it must always appear inadequate." The staff of the NHS, in myriad roles, is utterly committed to evolving and improving this unique organisation. Without daily micro and macro management of that service, that would not be possible.

Alongside the strides in medical science have come strides in medical management, helping to cast a more efficient, more effective protective net over our country. In 1900, 160 babies out of every 1,000 died before the age of one. The 1981 census shows that 11 babies in every 1,000 died before the age of one. Infant mortality rates have been transformed by vaccination programmes, better sanitation and improved standards of living. The NHS has been central to that heartening achievement. There is one final point to be made about the path the NHS has taken over the last 60 years and where its management has led it. Today, both men and women live an average of 10 years' longer than they did before 1948. Bevan's dream has become a reality. The rest is, perhaps, just detail.

Beyond the fence

THE TROUBLE WITH FENCES is that people sit on them. Or they stand on opposite sides of them, never quite seeing things from the other person's perspective. At times it must seem like there is one never-ending fence snaking its way throughout the NHS, with doctors on the left and managers on the right. The thing is, it's completely understandable.

Good management is about good communication, engaging with people, motivating them, leading from the front and getting them on board with decisions, ideas and change. Good medical practice is about ensuring the safe delivery of care to patients. Simple. If only it were, because the trouble is, there can't be many organisations as complex and convoluted as the NHS.

You've got government policies coming top-down. There's a deep and rooted sense of history running right through. Unlike the private sector, staff cannot be offered financial incentives for achievements. Solutions that might save money or speed up processes are fine in theory, providing they don't compromise the safe delivery of care in practice. And then there's the very real issue about who actually has the final say when it comes to changing the way medical practitioners practise. After all, consultants, nurses and anaesthetists all operate to standards, codes and guidelines set by their own Royal College, not the hospital.

"Oh, East is East, and West is West, and never the twain shall meet." Or perhaps not. What happens when one steps into the other's world, and they start to absorb each other's culture, ethos and learn another 'language'? How powerful can it be when doctors and managers bridge the gap and work together to improve services?

Dr Mark Johnston trained to become a doctor at St Andrews and Manchester. When he graduated in 2000 he went on to do surgical house jobs at Stepping Hill hospital in Stockport, and Blackpool Victoria hospital, before carrying out his basic surgical training at neighbouring Royal Preston, and gaining his membership to the Royal College of Surgeons. "I worked for six years to call myself doctor," he remembers, "and then another four years to call myself mister. It goes back to when surgeons were barbers and served an apprenticeship."

Yet despite all this serious investment in his career, in 2007 he decided to go into management. "I knew all my years learning and training would not be wasted in management because I would still be drawing on my clinical skills in terms of how I want to treat my patients, how I communicate and how I want services to develop," he says. "It's experiences like waking a consultant radiologist at 1am to request a CT scan for a patient who needs it. There is an art to that. I draw upon those experiences all the time. When I speak to clinicians, it's about being concise and getting straight to the point. Clinicians can switch off very quickly unless you speak their language. So all those skills have given me a head start in dealing with senior people as a manager."

The decision to switch from doctor to manager started with a job ad for a medical adviser in the strategic health authority (SHA) working around the European Working Time Directive. "It was a pretty big challenge. The directive becomes law for all doctors in 2009. Our chief executive wanted to do it a year early. There were a lot of challenges in terms of low junior doctor morale, following the problems with the new Medical Training Application System (MTAS, AKA Moving To Australia Soon). It is very difficult to get doctors to sign up to something before they have to, especially when it has the potential to affect their pay, but we have reached 95% plus, with only a few difficult specialist areas to go.

"For whatever reason, doctors only seem to listen to doctors. I have a much better rapport with consultants because they know I was a clinician. Looking back to the work I did at the SHA, the management team had been struggling for a long time to get engagement from doctors. But I had much more success in getting them on board and getting them to listen and engage. I feel we can improve service quicker than managers who don't always have the understanding of how clinicians think or what motivates them.

"But way before we got to this point with the programme, even in the first couple of weeks, I realised I wanted to be an NHS leader more than I ever wanted to be a doctor. I am now hell-bent on becoming a chief executive within the next nine years – no one can say I lack ambition. There is an untapped cohort of people below consultants who would be willing to leave their medical careers and pursue a career in management. In fact, several junior doctors have paid out of their own pocket to do MBAs."

Mark is currently the directorate manager of medicine at Blackpool Victoria hospital. "We have two directorates in the medical division, specialist medicine that I manage and acute medicine. It is my responsibility day-to-day is to ensure that all of my wards and all of my services are running as smoothly as possible. This includes things like the 18-week target and cancer targets. The key to this is translating these target improvements into language the clinicians would rather hear, improving outcomes. On top of that I have a host of service development plans where engaging the support of the consultants is essential.

"I want to improve dermatology, so I'm looking at what they are doing in another trust, which is thought to excel, to get an idea of best practice and new models of service. There is potential for improvement. Our stroke service has started to improve a lot, but I want to up the ante and become a national exemplar. And in terms of the elderly, we've cut down the length of stay and improved patient care on two wards. Now I want to roll that out across the trust; it's called the LEAN process."

Mark believes that many of the senior clinicians in the trust are "like sponges", in that, "they want to find out all about management. They realise they don't have all the skills but, historically, doctors don't like to admit they have weaknesses. Now they are saying: 'We would like to understand how to write budgets and business plans.' Trusts are no longer assuming that the oldest and most-respected consultant will make the best medical director or clinical director. They are looking at plucking out people who show real initiative. As a doctor, you are continually trying to get your junior doctors up to the next level in their career path. And that is something I want to bring into my management style."

And for proof, one has only to look at a two-day induction to the NHS Graduate Management Training Scheme that Mark and a colleague, Yasmin Ahmed-Little, were invited to speak at. "We did a stand-up 'Carry on Doctors and Managers' routine," he says. "I played the part of a consultant and Yasmin, who was the manager of the European Working Time Directive Team at NHS North West at the time, took the role of a middle manager. What we were trying to do was show the students, all 200 of them, the stereotypical 'I am God'-type consultant versus the typecast target- and budget-focused manager who doesn't care about patients.

"Yasmin was sitting on the stage behind a desk typing at a laptop, as managers do, when I burst in from the back in full scrubs, shouting and screaming at her about the planned closure of a theatre. She remained calm and I yelled at her something along the lines of: 'Well you can explain personally to all my patients because it is your fault.' She replied: 'I did try to get in touch with you about it but your personal assistant said you don't like to be disturbed on the golf course.'

"For the closing line, we both said: 'I want to improve patient care,' at the same time, and we looked at each other, surprised at the fact that we both wanted the same thing. It was a way of communicating that despite the different approach we are all on the same side.

"After we had embarrassed ourselves to death we split the room and highlighted what people think about managers and doctors. It was a word association game. I said 'doctor' and they said 'intelligent'. Then I said 'manager' and they said 'targets', 'budgets'. The idea was to get all those misconceptions out in the open and then to break them down and address them."

After the fun and games, albeit with a serious undertone, Mark and Yasmin did a presentation about the grades, roles and specialisms of doctors, focusing on the fact that they're not superhuman, but they are not monsters either. "They were quite surprised that until you get to the senior levels, doctors are relatively poorly paid even compared to management grades. So they are not these people flying round in sports cars. Then there's the European Working Time Directive, which we had just implemented in our SHA, which actually means less work, less pay.

"Communication is a two-way street: it's not just telling people what to do. Engage with them because they will come back and ask you questions, and the ones who do come back are probably the ones you will be able to work with and develop a relationship with as a manager in the future."

Meanwhile, some 300 miles away on the south coast, an unusual chemistry experiment is taking place on level seven of Derriford hospital in Plymouth, one of the largest general hospitals in Europe. The two elements involved are one group of senior doctors and another group of managers, and the lab is the offices of the hospital's service improvement team. All the evidence so far from this experiment suggests that putting these two together produces some very positive results.

With 6,500 staff and hundreds of patients, relatives and visitors milling around every day, Derriford hospital is the size of a small town. Since late 2006, five senior consultants have been regularly coming to a quiet corridor away from the daily human drama and hubbub to work as part of a team with six managers and their support staff.

In an unmistakable symbol of their joint approach, the two service improvement team leaders, Steven Allder, consultant neurologist and head of clinical systems engineering, and Debbie Taylor, head of service improvement, sit just three feet apart in a small, shared office. It's a measure of the distance they have travelled along an axis that has been described by one healthcare analyst as running between the two extremes of financial realism (managers) and clinical purity (consultants).

"The great thing about the team is that we have a shared understanding of the problems and challenges in the hospital," says Steve. "Debbie and I have a really natural, unthinking and intuitive relationship." Debbie adds: "The sole purpose of our team is to improve the quality of services and reduce costs. We can't do that without the clinicians and, actually, they do want to be involved. It is crucial that Steve and I work together. We are absolutely both singing from the same hymn sheet."

What is immediately obvious is that both have brought essential skills and capacity to the party: the managers bring their organisational and change management experience; and the consultants bring clinical insight into patient services and influence among the movers and shakers in the hospital – the senior doctors who can make service improvements happen.

James Hobbs is a manager on the team who has co-operated closely with Steve on achieving the four-hour target from a patient's arrival in A&E to either admission to the hospital or discharge. "Having Steve with us has made all the difference in terms of finding a joined-up way forward and getting clinical buy-in," he says. "Before we started working in this way, this was just seen as a management-directed target and everyone was disengaged. If we missed the target, people just saw it as the fault of A&E, rather than looking at the much more complex picture behind it."

Steve describes James as "my right-hand man on achieving the four-hour target". Working together, they have tracked A&E patients' pathways through the hospital and revealed the underlying reasons for the common afternoon bottleneck. "Although it was seen as something A&E needed to put right by themselves, we discovered the real reasons was beds were not being freed up for patients to be admitted for further treatment," notes James.

"Patients were not being discharged early enough in the day from our medical assessment unit, which is the patient's next stop after emergency admission." Steve offers the analogy of a hotel: "If the hotel management didn't get people to leave at 10am, how on earth would you get the room ready for the next guest?"

Steve and James know that if doctors are going to act, they need solid, reliable information on which to base their decisions. Having discovered the wider causes of delays in A&E, the team created some tailored solutions. One was to bring the ward consultant round an hour earlier, which meant that patients who were ready to be discharged were leaving earlier in the day.

A further innovation was a daily morning meeting of the medical assessment unit consultants with their specialist colleagues, allowing them to prioritise their ward rounds so they see patients who are ready to be discharged first. Logical maybe, but it couldn't have happened without some of the hospital's most senior doctors becoming convinced of the need for change.

That is where Steve's presence on the team is crucial. James explains: "It is so difficult for managers working on their own to build up that respect from clinical colleagues. Steve's involvement was really key in helping us to understand how clinicians' minds work, so we were able to present them with a convincing picture of what was happening and persuade them to make changes."

Now, James says, after two years of the joint team being in action in the hospital, he is beginning to see the culture changing all around him. "The consultant group I have worked with are coming up with ideas for further improvements all the time. They will ask me to come down and see what they are proposing and whether it is sensible, and I will support them with the information they need to take it further. The doctors are totally on board."

For his part, Steve says that working with the managers was, "in my own interests", because it helped him to get his hands on the levers of organisational change. "The managers have a much better understanding of the organisation and change that we need to get a grip of. They understand how change really works." He is happy to debunk the myth that, while managers have a nerdy addiction to data, analysis and targets, doctors are only interested in a 'pure' model of patient care, regardless of the financial implications.

"Once you show doctors the evidence, they really want to get involved. Consultants are highly qualified people, with two or three degrees, sometimes more. We are used to looking at evidence and we want to see it. When I showed my colleagues the evidence for what was happening with patient pathways, they could see the point immediately. They need to see a scientific approach, and they can be convinced. Once they were persuaded, they redesigned their own systems, and that's how we began to move towards meeting the four-hour target."

Steve and the team are already using the successful approach they employed to improve the admission of A&E patients to tackle other key challenges; and Steve believes it can be applied to many of the knotty problems that get in the way of delivering the best possible hospital services.

When he finishes his ward rounds and clinics, Steve goes to join Debbie in their office. With the support of the managers and his four consultant colleagues on the team, he gathers key data and sits over his computer, analysing the information and creating graphs. But this is no dry-as-dust number crunching; as it appears on his screen, each graph is telling a compelling story about where service improvements need to be made in the hospital.

He insists that managers must be a part of it: "If you are really committed to improving things for patients, you have got to work to break down the barriers between doctors and managers." He describes the attitude of doctors who are dismissive of managers as "a very unsophisticated way of seeing things," arguing that, "different skills and powers to make things happen reside in different people and parts of the hospital. You have got to pull them all together to create change and improvement."

Steve and Debbie envisage spreading their understanding of how service improvement happens beyond the departments they have worked with, to the whole hospital. "I would like to see all doctors and managers throughout the organisation with some of the skills and understanding we have," explains Debbie, "because it is everybody's responsibility and everyone needs to know how to do this."

Steve adds that the joint approach he has helped develop at his own hospital could and should be echoed throughout the NHS. "The NHS is in the midst of wide-ranging reform. Doctors are going to have to start applying their brains, which are considerable, to these problems. When they meet managers, they need to start asking: 'What organisational change can this person help me achieve?' My drive is really clear. The principles of the NHS being free at the point of contact and equitable are so worth fighting for. But, with the immense challenges for the NHS ahead, if we doctors and managers just stay in our own little boxes, it could be squandered."

Fences are great. If you're a farmer. But they're not so good in the health services because they mark boundaries, points of no access and separation. Even if we can't get rid of them completely, at least we should punctuate them with more gates. And that's exactly what Mark Johnston, Steven Allder, Debbie Taylor, James Hobbs and the other members of their teams are doing. Access all areas.

Making the ordinary, extraordinary

IT WAS THE bonfire party that did it. The managers at Lewisham hospital, where Stephen Langford had his first clerical job, were organising a fireworks display on an old hospital site. Stephen stood and watched the show and thought: "I could have done better than that."

It was then that he realised that management was about organising people and things well. Not making a meal of it, as those lighting the rockets that November night seemed to be, but knowing what you want to achieve and motivating others to come along with you. The insight propelled him into a career dedicated to managing health services. That week he applied for the NHS regional administration training scheme.

Stephen had joined the NHS straight from Leeds University. "It was 1982 and almost impossible to get even a bar job. Universities had cancelled the milk rounds, when employers came round to see you. I can remember clearly my flatmate and I being able to plaster the kitchen wall with the different ways people told us 'no thanks'." He was up to the sink before he got a 'yes' from the medical records department of Lewisham hospital.

He found he loved every minute of it, soaking up the variety and the community life of the hospital, and joining in the Christmas activities. In an emblem of the co-operative spirit he has been working to engender ever since, he clearly remembers junior doctors and managers all getting stuck in as a team to put on the Christmas panto, rehearsing and acting together.

The management training he started was built on a foundation of trainees gaining very broad experience. Stephen began what had become known as 'the cook's tour'. "You went round the whole of the health service and did a bit of everything. So I was a porter and went into theatres and pushed dead bodies around. I spent a week as a domestic cleaning a ward. God that was hard work. I was mopping the floor and serving meals and doing everything. There are pleasures too, because you get to chat to people, but it's hard.

"I still remember very clearly what those roles were. It gives you an understanding that is very important later on. Having empathy for the whole range of jobs and carrying it with you and it still being vivid, that is crucial when you are trying to make things happen in an organisation."

After getting experience in different care settings all over the NHS, Stephen became an assistant administrator at King's College hospital, one of London's most famous, and busy, hospitals. He was responsible for the switchboard operation, the communication nerve centre of the hospital. His job was to rip out the 1930s-style telephony system and replace it with a computerised one that routed calls electronically.

It was a monumental change, involving training every staff member in the hospital and rewiring the entire building. His training had hardwired into him the need to understand a system from the inside. "If you can picture it, they used to have a switchboard with lots of holes in and they plugged in wires to make the right connections and route calls. I remember working on it to get an idea of what it was and I found it hugely complex and difficult. The people operating it had to be very quick, and very skilled."

It was the mid '80s. Madonna was telling it to us 'Like a Virgin', the very first mobile phone was available for anyone with the strength to carry this new status symbol around… and the NHS was undergoing a controversial leadership revolution, with the introduction for the very first time of general managers throughout the organisation.

Stephen was one of the first of this new breed, with a new post at Dulwich hospital, managing the doctors and nurses on eight wards. It meant that, from a very early stage in his career, teamwork with clinicians was just the way Stephen did things. "I worked very closely with medical and nursing directors. We were ambitious for the NHS – we wanted to make care on our wards as good as it could be."

He also wanted to make sure the hospital recruited and hung on to excellent nurses. And he had a completely new way of doing this – the creation of a new ward where nurses were in charge. "We set up this brand new ward, called Byron Ward, where nurses were in charge of patients' care."

It was an idea that was way ahead of its time – threatening, in a way, to doctors who traditionally were in charge. Stephen knew that getting them on board was essential. It was, after all, a model that developed nursing skills, helped make the most of hospital resources, and provided excellent care for the right patients. "We made the case for the change. We talked to them individually and we worked with others who influenced them."

It was also an innovation that goes to the very heart of NHS management. "Working with clinicians: that is the key issue for managers. If you can put clinicians in the driving seat of change with a shared aim for services, you are on the right track. If you think you can do it yourself, you are on the wrong track. Services are delivered pretty much by clinicians. It's them, and their ability to deliver high quality services that makes it happen or doesn't.

"I have enormous regard for clinicians. We are in a people business and it is people who deliver it and receive it. Our job is to communicate what excellent services look like. That empowers individual clinicians to lead things they feel passionately about. Trying to knock something down is a waste of energy. It's far more powerful to build on good practice to make it better. The successful managers are those who enjoy working with clinicians and get a buzz out of it."

Stephen also gets a buzz out of innovation. Although he has been in the NHS for more than 25 years, he still seems to be able to look at services in a new way. He benefits from the freshness of always asking: what is the best way of delivering services to patients and helping staff do the work?

He had more chances to turn this drive into reality at North East London Strategic Health Authority, where his job was explicitly to transform services: it was in the job title, executive director of service transformation. He was part of a group in 2003 that was aiming to break out of the rut of providing healthcare during 'normal office hours'. They made some fantastic improvements, including dramatically extending GP hours. Two pilot practices managed to generate an extra 2,200 GP consultations and 3,200 nurse consultations in the first three months.

In a way, Stephen is always trying to look at himself with fresh eyes, too. He has always been trying to jump out of his own skin. It's one of the ways he keeps on developing as a person and a manager. Things like submitting regularly to the tough questioning of a business mentor – someone he met on a senior managers' course and took on to act as a sort of external conscience, constantly able to challenge him and his way of doing things. Or measuring himself up against the Myers-Brigg Type Indicator, a Jungian personality test. "I found out that on the J-P axis, I am far more J than P. J is someone who will not be swayed or distracted from implementing a plan. P is someone who is constantly taking in new information and evaluating it."

If the worst of J may be a bull-headed determination, then the worst of P is bending with every latest whim, like a reed in the wind. Stephen is striving to operate somewhere in between, as someone who provides a clear vision and the drive to get there, but can also take in and react to new information.

Not only having good ideas, but also being able to see through change is an essential quality in Stephen's present post as interim chief executive of Barking and Dagenham Primary Care Trust. He surveys his borough, and sees huge changes to the local car industry, to the mix of people because of rapid immigration and to local politics. "All these things have an impact on people's health. Services are not always set up in the right way for people who have moved in to the local community. So we are trying to develop urgent care centres and to extend the hours of GP services."

He is balancing this understanding of the people and the place with the need to transform the trust to meet the challenges of becoming a major commissioner of services. "It is everything from how well you work with local partners to the hard outcomes you get in terms of patient care."

What is the most important factor in leading an organisation with a £300 million annual budget and some 800 staff? "To want to be the best and to want the best for local people. No one got motivated by saying 'Come on, let's go out there and be ordinary. Let's go out and enthuse people with mediocrity.' If someone says an improvement will take 18 months, let's try and do it in six."

So what are the fundamental guiding principles of Stephen Langford, NHS manager? He loves the health service. He's been working in it all his life. He has huge respect for the skills of clinicians and nurses. He's intelligent and personable. He's more J than P, but he tries to be a little bit P, at least some of the time. He has never forgotten what it's like to do the coalface jobs in the NHS, even for just a week. And he never stops looking for a better way to do things, and to make things better for the patients who come through his door.

Learn, re-learn and unlearn

....

From: Abena Ssanyu
Sent: Monday, October 06, 2008 11:20 AM
To: Salma Yasmeen
Subject: Breaking Through

Dear Salma,

I got your name from Eden Charles who told me that you were among the first intake on the Breaking Through's Transformational Leadership Programme in 2007. I'm really interested in getting an insight into the programme from someone who has experienced it first-hand. Hence the reason Eden suggested I contact you.

I've read that the objective is to increase the diversity of the NHS workforce at director level through enhancing attendees' personal insight, emotional intelligence and ability to make powerful and creative interventions. As I understand it, the programme (which I've heard is pretty radical in its style and approach) aims to give participants the self-belief and awareness to function as transformational leaders within their own organisation; and that it's about empowering people to maximise their potential. As a 30-year-old, highly-ambitious black, African woman with a desire to make a real difference, Breaking Through sounds like it was designed with me in mind.

I was just wondering why you went on the programme and what you got of out it? Did it really increase your self-confidence and give you a greater sense of authority? What insights did you gain about your personal effectiveness and how you might improve it? Has it made you better at managing any prejudices you might have had? Are you able to find better solutions in some of the more complex situations? Overall, are you more aware of how you can, both personally and as part of a team, play your part in delivering services that are more beneficial and effective?

I hope you don't mind me contacting you out of the blue, and I'm really sorry to have bombarded you with so many questions, but when I heard about this programme I was really intrigued, and wondered if there might be a career path in a different direction for me.

I look forward to hearing from you.

Kind regards,
Abena Ssanyu

....

From: Salma Yasmeen
Sent: Wednesday, October 08, 2008 3:41 PM
To: Abena Ssanyu
Subject: Re: Breaking Through

Dear Abena,
Thank you for your email, which I read with great interest. Of course I'd love to give you the benefit of my experience. Luckily I

kept a journal during the programme, so it'll be a pretty easy exercise putting those thoughts, memories and feelings down onto paper. As the expression goes, I'm sorry this is so long but I didn't have time to make it shorter!

When the Transformational Leadership Programme came up I was delighted. It's a top managers' programme and looked really comprehensive. It was a little bit unknown, based on experiential learning, which really appealed to me. I needed to make sense of how I was behaving and responding, and how I was perceived, all in a safe environment where I could grow, because on the job you are catapulted into something and it's relentless.

To drive change you have to be committed and you have to be on it constantly. There isn't the comfort of an oasis where you can step back, think and learn. And I was prepared to re-learn and to unlearn things because I really did want to be the best at what I was doing. I had always found it difficult to work with people who held on to traditional ways of doing things. How did I engage people without leading to open conflict? That was what was going through my head when I signed up for the programme.

The programme itself is five weeks spread over five months. Some of it is in the King's Fund in London, which runs it, but we went all over the place: to Dartmoor, to residential centres in Devon, and to real-live trusts undergoing massive changes in Ireland. It really gave me a deeper insight and understanding.

The first day was at the King's Fund. I remember it well. We had been asked to make contact with somebody prior to the start of the programme. I walked into the room, feeling quite apprehensive. Actually, everybody looked apprehensive. I had made contact with an anaesthetist, and I was able to find her, so that helped. There was a whole mix of people there, and I was wondering who they were, what they did, what they wanted, what their hopes were. My hopes on that first day were that I would be able to learn more about me: how to be more effective in driving change in the NHS and working with a whole range of people, including people who didn't want to work with me. It's so hard to keep on creating meaningful change in the NHS; you have to give something of yourself all the time.

At that point I was really willing to look deeply into myself, at my values and beliefs, to allow me to take on more responsibility and influence. I was really open about that, and what I did for a living in working with mental health services was linked very closely to what my values are. So it was very transparent, very on show. When you are challenging inequality, you are wearing your values on your sleeve all the time.

Valerie James and Eden Charles were leading the programme, and all five weeks were so different and focused us on different aspects of ourselves. One of the weeks that will stay with me forever was the most challenging for me. It went to the heart of a lot of the things I was facing. It was about the relationship between yourself and the system in which you worked. That was an incredibly powerful week. It did bring me to tears.

The light-bulb moment for me was when Carla, a black speaker who came in to talk to us, spoke about how the system over a period of time had a dehumanising impact, often leaving individuals feeling invisible and simply surviving on a daily basis – not thriving, which is what one has to do to create meaningful improvement and change in the NHS. I realised at that moment that while my drive was for equality, often it was equality for myself that I was really fighting for. It really hit home and I realised I couldn't continue with just driving myself for change.

Throughout the programme we did a lot of small group work. We had to select groups and as we did so every week we were asked to really think very consciously about why we were selecting people. That really brought home to me our natural prejudices and preferences and biases. We had to think about how that related to the other groups on the programme. It really represented the world in which we worked – the systems, the health teams and the trusts.

That was incredibly powerful, and really helped me to see how the way individuals worked had a collective impact. Often, we blame the system for our frustrations, but the reality is that we are the system! The thing the programme did for me was getting me to reconnect with my compassion; compassion for those who did not see the need for change in the way I did.

I also learnt about holding balance. Sometimes we are disappointed in people above us, or the people we work with. But people are afraid of change, which may be frustrating for me, but I have to remember that they have positive qualities and strengths that I needed to continue to work with. It was about going back and getting over those barriers and getting over the 'them and us' feeling.

We did a live consultant exercise in Ireland. It started off with something we were familiar with, but this time we learnt to ask questions in an appreciative manner, not a critical one, and to get people dreaming. We looked at a huge merger of the PCTs and trusts in Ireland. A lot of people were feeling like casualties of change. When we spoke to people it was so powerful, we really were able to give them a chance to express their emotions and sense of apathy and powerlessness.

By the end of it, we were asking them, "What is one thing you could do to create change, and what is your ideal vision for this service?" We are not used to asking questions like that in the NHS. But you could see people coming up with all sorts of different, imaginative and challenging ideas. So we began to tap into their hopes and dreams and ideas.

We got very honest feedback on how people perceived us. I heard I was someone who was very committed to change, very passionate, but that that could also be read as someone who was quite pushy, someone who didn't always listen. So in my fight for equality, I was also excluding people. I took a really good look at myself, which people are afraid to do, and recognised that I was successful in some ways but there were challenges in other areas and I wanted to get past that.

After the programme had finished, I began to understand patterns of behaviour, and understand different services and teams in a different way. In those situations I was consciously going in with a different mind set.

For instance, going to a meeting with a consultant who I was fully aware saw the issue differently. Equally, he was suspicious of me as a manager trying to change the way he worked and operated. So we would enter into a dialogue from a position of misunderstanding and mistrust. Instead, I had to think that he equally wanted to improve things for his patients; he equally wanted to make systems better. So I went in and let him know I wanted to work with him. I recognised that he had done a lot of transformational work and that he was going to lead a lot of the change we needed to see in the future.

The programme revealed to me that all these things were happening at a deeper emotional level, and that this was incredibly important to working relationships.

Phew! I'm sorry I've rattled on, but I hope that you find some of what I've said interesting and insightful, and that it inspires you to enrol on the programme. If you do, I'd love to hear how it went.

Regards,
Salma

From: Abena Ssanyu
Sent: Monday, October 13, 2008 9:40 AM
To: Salma Yasmeen
Subject: Re: Breaking Through

Hi Salma,
Thank you so much for replying, and so vividly and eloquently, too. I read and re-read your email many times, just to try and put

myself in your situation. I found it fascinating.

I forgot to ask, though, what are you doing now? The reason I ask is that I noticed from your email address that you're at Tower Hamlets PCT. How long have you been there, and in what capacity?

I really look forward to hearing back from you.

Kind regards,
Abena

....

From: Salma Yasmeen
Sent: Tuesday, October 14, 2008 4:12 PM
To: Abena Ssanyu
Subject: Re: Breaking Through

Hi Abena,

Thanks for the email. I'm really pleased that you found my words and thoughts useful. Again, of course I'd be delighted to help out.

You're right, I am in a new job, in a new city; the programme gave me the confidence to risk that. Once it was finished I did lots of things. I left my family home in Huddersfield, I got married, I left mental health services in Bradford where I had worked for 10 years – all my networks, contacts, everything – and moved to London to take up the Marie Curie Delivering Choice Programme in Tower Hamlets PCT.

Tower Hamlets is a pilot site for this programme. Its main aim is to improve end-of-life services and care for those patients at the end of their life, and give them genuine choices. To do it well involves so many services and agencies – the local authority, London ambulance service, the commissioners, the acute hospital trust, the local hospices, care homes, the voluntary sector and the PCT.

That is my vision for the Marie Curie programme I am now

running: that people are truly engaged and that whether you are somebody who works in a care home, a consultant, a nurse or a service manager, you have a shared vision and must really work together to deliver that. It is about building on the best of what is happening in the NHS, rather than being critical and knocking things down. One of the most important things I learned is the importance of engaging people in that journey of hope.

It is incredibly challenging because historically people diagnosed with cancer are more likely to be able to access good palliative care, whereas for those with other illnesses or conditions, there are huge challenges even being able to define what the end-of-life stage is. There is very little palliative care for those with renal failure, cardiac patients and those with dementia, for example.

Our challenge is to get physicians to recognise end-of-life stages and to implement great care irrespective of their diagnosis, culture or their sexuality. It is everybody's right to have a dignified death. There is a lot of complexity involved for somebody to be able to die at home, and there is the need for health professionals to work with a whole host of agencies. You may have to make sure they have transport to get home, equipment at home, a proper bed, access to stairs, medication, district nursing services and social services, and adequate support for the carers. So there is a lot to co-ordinate.

So how am I putting what I learned into practice? Well I suppose it's about recognising from the outset that it is absolutely central to bring clinicians on board and to involve them. So the way we have designed the teams on the Delivering Choice Programme is that we have different clinical leads, rather than just a single team co-ordinator, and the conversations are happening at senior levels.

I am much more aware of the human aspect of what change might mean for people. I am also mindful that there are a lot of different perspectives out there, and I try to be truly open to those different perspectives. I am now operating as a manager in a transformed and transformative way. In those situations where I might have ended up in conflicts early on in a relationship, I am now much more flexible. I tap into their feelings, and respond differently so that we are able to move forward together, rather than meeting a block early on. I am someone who has always wanted to create change and transformation, and I am now careful not to inflame, alienate or exclude, but to make everyone feel part of it. I'm really bringing that into the world of management.

For me, the programme was so powerful that it really recreated what happens in the outside world. We had such a mad, crazy, one-off time in our lives. There wasn't a day that went past that we didn't have loads of fun and laughter. They were getting us to do all sorts of things.

One of the weeks they had us doing outdoor activities, but I really can't read a map. So we were out on the Devon moors with a compass and it was freezing. We had to get ourselves to different destinations and I think three hours later we were still in exactly the same spot deciding which direction was west and where east and south were. It was about relying on each other, drawing on our different strengths.

When I get in touch with people from the programme we often reminisce about that. It was such a one-off experience that you cannot really relay to someone outside. It was really profound, and the effects are ongoing. I am still having light-bulb moments!

Hope that helps, and please feel free to write again if there's anything else you'd like to know.

Salma

From: Abena Ssanyu
Sent: Thursday, October 16, 2008 10:16 AM
To: Salma Yasmeen
Subject: Re: Breaking Through

Hi Salma,

Me again. Last time, I promise!

You mentioned that you used to work in mental health services. It's a very different field to the one I work in, but if you've got the time I'd be really interested to hear a bit about your path into the programme as one of my best friends is doing a postgrad diploma in mental health nursing at Sheffield Hallam University.

Sorry to take up even more of your time, but I always find that when I hear stories first-hand, they are always so much more memorable and personal.

Thanks.

Abena

From: Salma Yasmeen
Sent: Monday, October 20, 2008 11:36 AM
To: Abena Ssanyu
Subject: Re: Breaking Through

Hi Abena,

No problem, honestly. I actually find this pretty therapeutic.

My career in the NHS started as a mental heath nurse. Having qualified in Huddersfield, I took up my first post as a staff nurse on an acute ward in a mental heath hospital. I then moved on to working in the community, as that is where my interests really were. I was a nurse in Bradford with the Home Treatment Service (HTS), working my way up to team leader. I worked very closely with Professor Patrick Bracken, the team's consultant psychiatrist. I don't know if you've heard of him, but he's renowned for his work with the NHS as a clinical director, and is author of a number of books. Within the HTS we developed a philosophy of care that did not privilege the medical model but rather looked at understanding the cultural, economic and political issues in people's lives as being central to framing their experiences of mental heath and distress.

The Home Treatment team was one of the first in the country, and the main aim was to provide genuine choice for people with acute mental health issues, so that they could remain in their own homes rather than having to be admitted to hospital. We were dealing with people with post-natal depression, schizophrenia and those who were at risk of suicide; all the major acute mental health problems that would normally lead to being admitted to a ward. This service won a Beacon award from the Department of Health, which recognises outstanding achievement and excellence in particular areas of service delivery or community leadership. That was an extremely rewarding experience.

I left there in 2002 and led the development of a pilot initiative that later became a mainstream voluntary service in mental health called Sharing Voices Bradford (SVB), working alongside consultants. Aimed at people with mental health issues in BME communities, it was very successful. We thought we would do something radically different and engage people from diverse communities to begin to articulate and define their own understanding of mental health and illness, and explore what their solutions were. Then we wanted to see how they would work with commissioners and providers to create the services they needed. Within two years, this went from being a pilot service to an independent registered charity with its own premises in the heart of inner city Bradford. It took off that quickly.

The whole relationship between BME communities and mental

health services is one characterised by suspicion and mistrust. But with Sharing Voices Bradford we managed to engage local people to find out what they wanted. It led to services that were nothing like the traditional model. Service users did completely new things like setting up poetry, music and women's groups. Some people wanted sport as a way out of their mental health problems, so we challenged local sports and recreation services and succeeded in getting service users access to gym clubs. One young man who had a mental health diagnosis went on to qualify as a fitness instructor. That was a real result for him.

All this was a world away from medication and counselling, which are what these types of service have traditionally offered. We were not anti-medication or counselling, but simply believed that a bigger programme of support was needed. When people are distressed, what they need is hope, and that comes from many sources; from friends, family, from accessing social networks, from religion and places of worship. Some people need spirituality. Others need work opportunities and some need strong family relationships. Mental health issues are often intertwined with many of these issues. You have to have the vision of a brighter, sunnier, happier future, so our job was to broker more positive relationships between BME communities and the wider services. The project then became mainstream and was taken on and funded by the PCT.

At that point, we met Lord Kamlesh Patel, who was developing a comprehensive plan for BME communities to tackle the inequalities they experience. He was appointed by the secretary of state to act as national strategic director for the National Institute for Mental Health (England), charged with developing and implementing that organisation's Black and Minority Ethnic Mental Health Programme. SVB now has over 10 staff and continues to work with communities, commissioners and service providers, locally and nationally.

His strategy had three building blocks. Firstly, engaging community, so that they are involved in service planning and demystifying mental health and services. Secondly, developing appropriate and responsive service. And thirdly, using data intelligently. We actually added a fourth one, which was about developing the workforce so it was representative. It was all very exciting, particularly as this was the first time ever in the history of mental heath that the Department of Health had launched such a comprehensive policy initiative to tackle historical inequalities in mental heath. Perhaps what was most exciting was the role assigned to BME communities and the importance of their involvement and engagement in any change.

Then, in 2007, I became the Focus Implementation Site project manager for Bradford. FISs were pilot sites for the implementation of the Department of Health policy for BME services 'Delivering Race Equality in Mental Health'. We were trying to fast-track the implementation of the national strategy in order to improve mental health services for BME communities. It was incredibly challenging, not just in terms of trying to get commissioners, providers and service users to work together to develop a shared vision, but also in just trying to get everyone around the same table so that multiple perspectives genuinely informed change in the area of mental health. There was some real progress being made as a result of this and evidence of better engagement with BME communities and services. There is still a lot more to do but I was really excited and pleased with the level of progress and change. It was at this point in my career that I became aware of Breaking Through. And the rest you know.

If there's anything more you'd like to know, just ask. And please do write back to me with your experiences of the programme if you decide to go for it. I'd be really interested to see if you find it as much of an eye-opener as I did.

All the best.
Salma

From: Abena Ssanyu
Sent: Tuesday, October 21, 2008 7:13 PM
To: Salma Yasmeen
Subject: Re: Breaking Through

Hi Salma,

Yet more food for thought. Thank you so much.

My friend Rosemary has actually met Prof. Pat Bracken a couple of times, and says he's a real inspiration.

I will definitely be applying for the 2009 intake, and I'll let you know how it all works out.

Once again, thank you so much for your time.

Abena

Smoke trail

FAILURE. It's not a pleasant word. Or is it? To some it spells the end of something. To others, the start of something new. But what does it take to turn around an initiative that is perceived as failing? What are the keys to a manager and management making a real and lasting difference?

Neda Hormozi was, until recently, the tobacco and smoking lead for Hammersmith and Fulham PCT. She is now director for leadership development at NHS Interim Management and Solutions (IMAS), a body that pulls together managers with proven expertise so they can support NHS organisations that ask for help with a specific project or to tackle a problem.

IMAS also aims systematically to develop seasoned managers to lead change. It's a neat circle in Neda's life in a way, because when she joined Hammersmith and Fulham, it was less of an ordinary career move and more a brave bid to take on a serious new challenge.

"I started when the smoking target was one of their main key performance indicators and they had failed on it drastically. At the time, PCTs were star-rated and it was set so that if they didn't reach it two years running, they would lose two stars. They had already lost one star. They wanted someone to come in and turn it around, to help them hit the target."

Her professional background was originally in publishing and printing, despite having qualified as a chemist and been a post-doctoral researcher at King's College, London. Neda's experience gave her a solid grounding in business and organisational skills, but increasingly she felt less fulfilled by what she did. "I had reached a point in the private sector where it was all about the bottom line, and I wanted to do something that helped people and changed people's lives."

Smoking was an issue that Neda felt passionately about. "Smoking? I absolutely loved it. Imagine the best experience you've ever had. If you can top it up, that's what smoking was to me." She gave up after 20 years as a smoker thanks to a self-help book. "I have friends who still can't believe I don't smoke, because I would smoke under any condition: I would light up in the pouring rain, or straight after having a tooth out."

Her personal experience meant that she was highly motivated and energised by her new role. "Because I was an ex-smoker I wanted to put something back – for something that I had found so hard to do myself. It was just at the point where the debate had started about taking England smoke-free. I just felt my contribution would have an impact on people's lives. It was a massive transition for me, actually giving up quite a comfortable and senior job in the private sector to take on this new challenge."

Having made the courageous decision to follow her heart and make a difference, Neda was faced with a line of hurdles in her new role. "I've always been good at putting a lot of energy into things. Whatever it takes, I will get on and do it. The PCT had outsourced the (anti-smoking) service, but the organisation was not delivering. I realised we were doing really badly but there was a lot of fear in the PCT that if we did anything else we might do even worse. So we were frozen. I went to my boss, the director, and said, 'We're commissioning this service out and we have got to put a stop to it.' And she replied, 'But we're getting 100 quitters a year, if we lose these guys [the outsourced service] we won't even have them.'"

Turning the situation around was going to take vision and determination. "There were different elements to my strategy. Basically smokers are people who are more likely to get gum disease, or flu. So my first points of call were the GPs and the dentists. I had to make all of these front-line services, and others within the PCT, aware of the help available for smokers to stop.

"The other thing was getting in touch with the tobacco control network, because this was a national programme and I wanted to find out what support already existed. I knew there should be a lot out there. And there was. So I started linking into them – there were networks for the regions, there were particular groups to help Muslims with Ramadan, and all sorts of support networks. There was no budget because we'd used it all outsourcing to this organisation that wasn't delivering, so I couldn't even have an administrator. I remember spending until 8pm on new year's eve packing info into envelopes for GP practices about the stopping smoking services."

Coming from a business environment meant that Neda was not afraid to learn lessons from other success stories to give her a competitive edge. "The only way to do something well is to see how other people are doing it. So we built links with other PCTs which were hitting their targets, to find out how they'd done it. The first thing I learnt was that we needed a bigger team. Also, other people were having problems with the organisation we contracted out to, so I was able to go to my director with this which provided the confidence to stop outsourcing the work."

The next issue was the bottom line, an area whose importance Neda recognised and was adept at manipulating due to her previous private sector roles. "Agree a budget with the PCT for the work, that was the first step, based on the work that others were doing. So I came up with a plan based on all the best practice out there. The director of finance went through my business plan and doubled my budget. I actually ended up with one of the healthiest budgets in London for stopping smoking.

"As I contacted the regional networks, I was also contacting the local authority, acute trusts and businesses. Within the local authority, there was someone who was very keen to get support to help their staff. So we shared the budget there to get advisers for their staff. I was pulling in money from other organisations to expand the work and we also pulled in half a million pounds from the local authority to work specifically with women of child-bearing age."

Neda also recognised how essential it was to get help from other people. "I got support for what I was doing from very senior people – such as the director of innovation – who backed up my budget to the local authority. So I didn't do it all myself. You can't do these things by yourself." The fruits of her labour bore gratifying results.

"I reached a point where I had other colleagues in PCTs calling me and asking 'How are you doing this work?' I guess a big part of what I did was to identify the people who were doing great work. There was one woman in London who's a midwife and helps expectant mothers and has built a reputation for being one of the best advisers. She was in my patch, I came across her and she didn't let me go. I was using all the best people in the field. When I find good people, I work with them. And there are loads of good people in the NHS. It started to build an enormous momentum. We started to build a team of individuals who were putting in their own time to help the service grow and were all in place when I left."

So how do her experiences in the private and public sector compare? "The Department of Health sets us targets, because that's a way to get a movement started. The targets are a pain in themselves, but without them less would happen and move. It's only because of these targets that budgets get assigned and a new piece of work doesn't get forgotten in the usual run of business. The NHS, if you were to compare it to the private sector, would be a series of holding companies, each with its own budgets, its own target. You need these targets from the top as a spur to action, to pull the whole thing together."

Hammersmith and Fulham have now hit their smoking cessation targets for three years running. "In the first year we were just short of 800 smokers [quitting]. What was most gratifying was being involved in the whole smoke-free agenda. I bumped into somebody on the Tube recently who was in one of my first ever clinics and he said he hasn't had a cigarette since. I was just sitting there minding my own business and he thanked me. England is the only country in the world that has had a national stop smoking service. That is really something to be proud of, to shout about."

The key to Neda's success lay in her passion for the work, her belief that the initiative could be turned around, her ability to see what needed to be done and how to achieve it, and the skills' base she brought with her from her private sector job. The result benefitted her, the PCT and hundreds of former smokers. Failure is just a state of mind.

- Britain has been recognised as the European leader in tobacco control.
- In the 60 years since 1948, we have gone from a nation of smokers to one where smoking is viewed in the main as an anti-social habit.
- In 1948 in Britain, 82% of men and 41% of women smoked: by 2005, it was 24% of the population.
- Since the Smoke Free England legislation in July 2007, 235,000 people have given up with the support of NHS Stop Smoking services.
- A smoker is four times more likely to give up successfully with the support of NHS services.

Handled with care

FREEDOM. Quality of life. Choice. Independence. As commissioners, primary care trusts (PCTs) now hold the purse strings and therefore have considerable power at their fingertips. When that power is used to effect direct benefit to patients, the results are little short of miraculous. Take the case of one patient suffering from Chronic Obstructive Pulmonary Disease (COPD) in Swindon. Thanks to improvements in the way the PCT organised services around people, the patient was able to go away on holiday for the first time in years. Or the 98-year-old woman in Hillingdon, north London, who had breathing difficulties but was still able to stay in her own home – where she wanted to be – rather than having to be admitted to hospital. And all because of a new team set up by the PCT to offer crisis care for up to 48 hours in the patient's home.

Now, as head of the NHS talent pool Interim Management and Support (NHS IMAS), Antony Sumara is developing a cadre of seasoned leaders to drive improvements in the NHS. He has been the chief executive of several organisations including Heart of Birmingham PCT and Hillingdon PCT. The first covered a very deprived population; the latter was working to overcome a financial deficit. In both, Antony helped reshape services, moulding them around patient needs. "PCTs need to remember always what they are there for," he says. "When I was with Heart of Birmingham PCT, our offices were just across the road from the public health offices. Every day I used to see this poor guy who was obviously mentally ill – he used to mutter and spit. A lot of people thought he was objectionable, but my view was 'It's my job to make him well'. It's the single thing that drives me.

"PCTs have got a fantastic opportunity to make a massive difference to patients. It's about how you get the best out of every pound you spend. It should be about meeting the needs of the patient; and the PCT is closest to the patient. Hospitals provide a great service, but patients don't want to be in hospital. What they want is a good hospital when they are ill. PCTs need to focus on keeping people well and out of hospital. We need to set up services in the way that achieves that."

While chief executive of the Heart of Birmingham PCT, Antony was involved in reshaping its diabetic services, moving a lot of patient care out of hospitals and into GP surgeries. It was one of the biggest transformations in the country, taking around 5,000 outpatient attendances out of the system over a two-year period. "People were going in to hospital clinics in their thousands," he remembers. "The clinics were overcrowded. So we took GPs through a process, saying 'Could you provide this sort of service in the surgery and what skills would you need to do that?' We worked very collaboratively with the consultants in the hospital because they are the experts, and the last thing we want is to undermine a hospital or throw it into crisis with the changes we are making. You need good hospitals!"

The PCT put together a training programme for the GPs with Warwick University. "More than 100 GP practices took up our opportunity, and they transformed things for diabetic patients." GPs started to work together, talking through issues with each other, more nursing time was put in place and eight advanced practitioners from the US were recruited. "This was so much better for patients. You are not one of 40 people sat in a clinic. You are with a GP who knows your history, your family and you get regular check-ups. Patients only got referred to a consultant if they were less stable, which was less often because they were being looked after much better."

Antony was with Heart of Birmingham for about four years. When he arrived at Hillingdon PCT at the end of 2006, it was £87 million in debt and losing £25 million a year. "They had services in place to keep people out of hospital and in the community," he says. "But they hadn't invested enough to make sure it was working. We are accountable to the public. They pay our wages. I am very proud and very clear about that. It's not my money."

Some of the very positive things the trust was doing included a nurse-led rapid-response team that offered crisis care in a patient's own home for up to two days and two nights, preventing hospital admissions. The senior nurse running the team, Sue Elvin, estimated in 2006 that they were managing to prevent nearly 80% of the people they saw from being admitted to hospital. Part of Antony's approach to get Hillingdon back in the black was to correct accounting errors and make sure community services like these were properly funded, helping the PCT to cut its hospital bills each year and preventing the weak finances that can lead to community services being underfunded, more patients in hospital and the consequent spiral of decline. While he was there, the trust also began negotiations with its GP surgeries to open an urgent care centre, providing an alternative to hospital A&E for patients with minor problems.

Although Antony has worked at the highest levels of the NHS for many years, in conversation he does not sound like a chief executive – or perhaps he does sound like the best sort of chief executive. Not pompous, nor self-approving, but radical and passionate. He notices the little things – the piece of rubbish on the hospital floor, the elderly patient, whose nightclothes were rucked up, compromising her dignity. A colleague of his says: "Antony is all about the patient. With him, it's patient, patient, patient."

What is behind this unshakeable focus? A patient is a person at their most vulnerable, so perhaps a clue comes from his parents' background, both of whom were Polish refugees and who were forced to work in German labour camps across Czechoslovakia, Italy and Russia during World War II. They were reunited in 1945 and were in Italy when the liberating forces arrived – their first child was born on the ship to the UK. Antony was their fifth and last child, born in a hut, part of a short-term housing complex for refugees in Whitchurch.

Antony was only 18, and studying at university, when he got his first NHS job, working part-time as a nursing auxiliary in a hospital for the elderly and people with head injuries. "There I was, the 18-year-old son of Polish refugees working with these West Indians who are some of the best people I have ever met. They taught me everything I know about caring for patients." And it's absolutely clear that that attitude is still very much with him today.

From an entirely different background, Sarah Chalmers, acting urgent care network manager for Bath, North East Somerset, Swindon and Wiltshire Health Community, and who went through the Graduate Management Training Scheme, shares a remarkably similar outlook. Swindon PCT is in the final stages of achieving full integration with the social care team in Swindon Borough to deliver services that cross traditional boundaries, such as GP-led services for the homeless and 'telehealth' services for vulnerable patients with long-term health conditions.

"Social care and health have a lot of co-responsibility," she says. "A patient with social care needs often has health needs. Fortunately, Swindon PCT is coterminous with the borough. We realised that the only way to deal with the patient as a whole person was to work much more closely together and to have social workers on discharge teams and to share commissioning space. We have a PCT commissioning team and they share an office with their colleagues in social services. We sit together, asking questions, learning about the other service's perspective. It is far easier for me to walk across to someone else's desk than to set up a meeting. And there are things that are blindingly obvious to a social worker that I wouldn't think of and vice versa."

She cites as an example an injury common when elderly people suffer a fall, a fractured neck of femur. "They are going to need treatment for the fracture, physio and occupational therapy. This is a joint responsibility of health and social care. Social workers can contribute an understanding of the assessments that the council needs to make to adjust the home environment, provide stair rails, grab rails and so on, and how to go about providing home helps."

An innovation that is providing enormous patient benefits right now is 'telehealth', a machine with a computer, attached to which is a set of scales, a modem, a blood pressure cuff, a blood-oxygen (SAT) machine and a blood-glucose monitor. It doesn't end there. At a pre-set time the machine will ask the patient or their carer if they're feeling well and whether, for instance, they've taken their inhaler today. To which, the patient answers "yes" or "no". That information is then emailed to a call-handling centre where a nurse assesses how well the patient is managing their condition, and how they are faring. If the patient is fine, nothing happens. If the patient's parameters are worrying, a nurse will visit and offer health advice. Alternatively, the patient can call their GP at any time, and instead of simply saying "I feel a bit poorly", the GP can see 10 days' worth of readings. "We reckon it pays for itself in one avoided admission," adds Sarah. "We trialled it with COPD, but it worked so well that we have now expanded it to patients with congestive heart failure and diabetes." And it was thanks to the simple innovation of 'telehealth' that one COPD patient during the trial period gained the confidence and the ability to manage the condition that allowed him for the first time in years to leave home for a short break away.

Sarah is keen to point out that, while part of her job is promoting the 'telehealth service', it was already in place when she arrived as a manager at Swindon and is one of the Trust's nurse-led initiatives. But the reason she is so passionate about it is that it brings such huge benefits for patients themselves. "Obviously there are always going to be silos, but there is a real ethos here that you put the patients in the middle of it and you work the services around it. In other places you hear things like 'well if social services did their job then we could do ours'. You don't hear that here because everyone is working together. Swindon is very patient-focused. There is really strong, high-level management that isn't precious and really does value working across service boundaries. There is a lot of scope for knowing each other personally and knowing people's faces. They value personal relationships and training. After all, if people didn't get ill, develop medical complications or have accidents, we wouldn't need PCTs in the first place.

"I think there is a real culture here of informal shadowing and speaking to each other. It makes all the difference. The changes are built into the highest levels of management. All the directors are joint appointments, so it irons out a lot of the management and accountability issues. People go to the same meetings and there is much more scope for people to be able to free up time for issues that need to be tackled because it is coming from the same leaders."

Patients in the main don't care about the 'wiring' behind the services they use. As Antony says, most of them probably don't even know what a PCT is. What matters is that the PCT is there, behind the scenes, working in whatever way is best, but always remembering what it is there for.

Ideas in action

ONCE TWO STICKS were just two sticks. Then someone thought differently about them, rubbed them together and changed the course of human history. Obviously not all ideas have such profound effects, but even small changes can create big improvements: they can speed up activities, increase efficiency, promote harmony, reduce costs and, most importantly, save lives. Things are often done the way they're done because that's the way they've always been done. That doesn't necessarily mean it's wrong; yet neither does it mean it's right. So move your mind just an inch or two to the left and grab another perspective; stand on mental tip-toes and look down on something rather than directly at it; and if a process, system or chain of events feels like it can be made to work better, then it probably can.

Ideas make the world go round. In fact, it was because someone questioned the accepted thinking of the day that we actually discovered the world was round. But even the most brilliant ideas have no currency in the real world unless someone acts on them, delivers them and manages them. That's how things get better, for patients, for staff, for the entire health system. That's how progress happens. That's how the NHS moves forward.

THE OUTLOOK'S BRIGHT IN CORNWALL

What do weather forecasts have to do with cutting hospital admissions in Cornwall? The answer is that scientists at the Met Office in Exeter have found that interpreting the patterns of the isobars can help keep patients with lung conditions healthier and out of hospital.

Sudden cold snaps trigger an increase in hospital admissions among people with chronic obstructive pulmonary disease (COPD). Because of this, the Met Office has been working with Finnish healthcare software specialist, Medixine, to develop an early warning system called 'Healthy Outlook®'. Trialled in Cornwall during winter, the results were quite staggering: emergency admissions of COPD patients to hospitals were cut by an incredible 52%.

The health forecasting system uses the Met Office's supercomputers to spot wintry weather coming and trigger an automated call to patients whose lungs might be adversely affected, giving them essential advice on how to keep themselves healthy. They can then take the simple step of staying indoors, making sure they have enough food and medical supplies to see them through the temperature drop. This 'precautionary' period can last for 10–12 days after the cold weather sets in.

In the Cornish trial, nearly 500 COPD patients subscribed to the service, meaning that during the winter these people received calls from the automated system and answered questions about how they were faring and whether they needed repeat prescriptions. Their answers were fed through to their GP surgeries the next day via a web link. The system worked so well that during the following winter, others surgeries across the country joined up to the scheme – in all, more than 8,500 patients in 160 GP practices.

So what could the potential impact be? There are around one million patients who have been diagnosed with COPD in the UK, and they account for one in eight emergency hospital admissions. That's a million bed days at a cost of £250 million each year. As part of the service, patients receive an information pack at the start of the season giving them information about their condition and what to do to help keep them well. Personalised automated calls are then delivered from October to March as the environmental conditions dictate. The money-saving potential of the service across the NHS is huge, and the health team at the Met Office is researching other conditions where weather plays a role.

SOARING EMERGENCY RESPONSES SET ALARM BELLS RINGING

The sound of an ambulance siren is both frightening and reassuring. Frightening because someone, somewhere, must be in trouble. Reassuring because you know that someone is on the way to help. The problem is, it costs £200 a time to send an ambulance out – more if a patient is taken to hospital or admitted to a ward and with an ageing population (the number of people over 65 increased by 31% between 1971–2006) and more people living with chronic conditions (15 million in England), the number of call-outs is continually rising.

But not for the South Central Ambulance Service, where patient report forms, which are completed by paramedics after each emergency response, are scanned into the Clinical Audit Reporting System (CARS). The data is then used to audit and improve clinical performance so that services are working much better for patients who use them. CARS can be used to pinpoint patients who frequently call 999, but whose health could be improved if they had access to alternative services in the community. It shows where emergency responses take place, such as the address of an individual patient or a particular area or building, giving vital clues as to how resources can be better used.

For example, the system showed that one 65-year-old patient

had made 54 calls in seven months because of chest pains. And on 54 occasions, an ambulance went out (at £200 a go, do the maths). An appropriate package of primary and community care was put in place, resulting in zero emergency calls from the patient over the next six months. In another case, an 82-year-old diabetic patient was found to have made 24 emergency calls in four months. Following the introduction of a care package, this also went to zero in the next five months. And it's not just about individuals. CARS also showed that there had been 60 ambulance call-outs to a nightclub for assaults and alcohol-induced emergencies in 12 months. Evidence from the ambulance service was used in court and, as a result, conditions were put on the club's licence, while new management was also installed. Over the course of the next 12 months, the number of emergency responses was reduced by 90% – to just six incidents.

It has long been said that 'information is power'. This proves the point emphatically. Not only that, but when data is used intelligently, it can save money and ensure that the ambulance resource is on hand for those who really do need it. North East Ambulance Service NHS Trust also has a system called Pathways, which uses the triage system for all 999 calls, allowing the team to identify how urgent a call is and refer it to other services rather than send an ambulance unnecessarily. Other primary care trusts and commissioners are exploring other ways to identify gaps in provision and unmet patient needs.

ROBOPHARMACY

Norfolk and Norwich University Hospital NHS Foundation Trust is one of many hospitals that is improving services through automation. A robotic dispensing system has enabled it to re-engineer the pharmacy service and release expert pharmacy staff to directly support nursing and medical staff on the wards, while also reducing turnaround times for medicines.

When we say robot, we're not talking R2-D2, Sonny in 'I Robot' or Mechagodzilla, we're talking about a big box that has four bays, in each of which are a number of shelves set at different heights. The old system worked like this: a pharmacist would store the drugs in alphabetical order, with enough space in between so that he or she could reach in and take out whichever pack or container they needed.

The new robotic system works thus: a stock of drugs is fed into the robot and stored wherever there is a space to fit the boxes. Think of it like a hard drive on a computer that finds the space and fits it in where it can. By using robotic arms, which suck out the packets, 45,000 boxes can be safely stored, with the software showing where the drug can be located.

So when a prescription comes in, a dispenser will type in the prescription details; the software will then link into the robot and say "I need a box of paracetamol for Mrs Bloggs"; the robot will access where it is, retrieve it and put it on a conveyor belt which will send it down a chute to the dispensing pharmacist who will label it. The result: more pharmacists are able to stand by doctors on the ward rounds, where they can make the most of their expertise, and where they can pass on their knowledge about the optimum use of drug therapies to junior members of the clinical team. What is more, patients are getting their medicines faster.

The system also helps with ward boxes because staff can put in a list of all the drugs needed and the robotic dispenser will pick these automatically off the shelves. This can be done out of hours, if necessary, allowing staff to be used more efficiently and effectively. Plans for the future include adding additional software so that the robot can carry out the labelling, which will allow staff to dial in overnight and dispense a drug over the phone during emergencies or out of hours dispensing.

PUTTING THE FOOT DOWN ON EMISSIONS

As Europe's single biggest organisation, the NHS produces around a million tonnes of carbon every year. To meet its target for 2050, it aims to cut this by at least 600,000 tonnes. One way is to reduce the environmental impact of the 15.5 billion passenger miles travelled each year by staff and patients. How?

In Cambridgeshire, the answer lies in the introduction of 'H1', the Addenbrooke's bus, the first public bus service in the country to be commissioned and managed by the NHS, and recognised nationally as an exemplar for travel plans. The Cambridgeshire hospital, reported to be the largest single generator of traffic in the county, was highly commended in the National Transport Awards (the 'Oscars' of the transport industry) in the category of 'Business Contribution to Sustainable Transport'.

In another first, Addenbrooke's also offers staff interest-free loans to buy pushbikes or mopeds, 16 rideshare cars and discounted weekly bus tickets. Together, these initiatives have reduced car usage by more than a fifth and increased bus and bicycle journeys by 13% and 4% respectively. Around half the hospital staff now take the bus or cycle to work. And the air in Cambridgeshire is a little bit cleaner.

INSPIRING AND BEING INSPIRED BY THE COMMUNITY

Problem: in an area in north east London there are a growing number of people from minority communities who are socially excluded, cut off from mainstream services because of cultural, language or other barriers. It means that thousands of people (many of whom have long-term conditions or disabilities) miss out on essential health services and care. Clearly this is not good for them, and for service it means the health inequalities they hope to tackle get worse. From a health management perspective, this situation also reduces the effectiveness of the resources available for the local population.

Thinking: create a cadre of people from within ethnic minority communities to signpost the way for these patients to access and use services.

Solution: the Health Guides Project, a collaboration between the local NHS, a voluntary organisation called Social Action for

Health, and local communities. It aims to tackle the health consequences of social exclusion by helping patients access services by giving them information and guidance in their own language, promoting self-care and self-management, relieving bottlenecks in the system that result from misinformation about how to access services, understanding people's experiences of accessing services and engaging them in deciding how they want to use services.

Health guides are local people from a growing range of minority communities (such as Bengali, Somali, Congolese, Caribbean and Kurdish), trained and supported by NHS project workers to help others in their community improve their health and access local services. They run community-based, own-language group sessions to address people's healthcare issues and concerns; represent local people and feed back what they think to health and social care organisations; guide patients in accessing the services they need; promote health and wellbeing; and help people to take a greater role in managing their own health conditions.

Not only has the initiative succeeded in achieving its aims, but it has also breathed life into the employment prospects of community members who trained as health guides, with half of the 75 finding work within six months. Due to the enormous response to the original posts advertised, the project was also extended to include mental health service users.

As this chapter demonstrates, the NHS is absolutely alive with new ideas; metaphorical lights going on all over the place, each one helping to illuminate the future a little more clearly. Take the surgical team at Great Ormond Street hospital who watched videos of the Ferrari and McLaren pit stop teams to get ideas for improving the complicated handover process from the operating theatre to intensive care. Or University College hospital, London, which has developed an infection-resistant keyboard that it is using in its high dependency units, where patients are especially vulnerable. Or Imperial College's project 'Second Health', which represents the health service within the virtual reality game 'Second Life'. In it, a leading clinician appeared as a mermaid and addressed 200 of her peers in a virtual international surgery conference before taking questions in real time. It is currently being developed for people who cannot attend real events. All brilliant. But only when they are actually brought to life. And that's where managers come in, both in the real and the virtual world.

Thought leading

TYPE THE QUESTION 'what makes a good leader?' into Google and you'll get around 21,000,000 results in less than a tenth of a second. Suffice it to say, it's an enormous topic with a wealth of perspectives, articulations and interpretations; some highly perceptive, some rather obvious, others little short of nonsense. To try and cut through the clutter and make some sense of it all is a highly complex, perhaps even impossible, task. The truth is there is no single, foolproof method of creating great leaders. But there are ways of equipping people with the tools that can help.

And that is precisely what Valerie James is doing through her focus on helping leaders and organisations understand and manage conflict and change, creatively. She directs programmes for the King's Fund, an independent charitable foundation that works for better health. The first programme is called Transformational Leadership and is all about transforming managers into leaders so that they can then go out and effect transformation in their part of the NHS. A second, Management for Specialist Registrars, is for registrars who are about to make the step up to consultant. In this programme she challenges them and tackles their prejudices about managers so that they can collaborate more creatively in the future. The important thing about the approach Valerie has developed with these programmes is that she is getting people to open their minds, and, in the process, she is helping develop the sort of creative and open-minded leaders we need in the NHS.

Put simply, Valerie's role, mission even, is to help nurture the future leaders of the NHS. Now that is some challenge, which she meets by looking at the person as a whole, not only giving them insights into the complexities of the organisation, but also focusing on the complexities of their own make up, and how that impacts upon their interactions with others. She develops people's emotional and political literacy, making them far more aware of their unconscious motivations and, as a result, far more effective leaders.

"If you watch 'Casualty,'" she says, "you'll see an administrator character lurking around, a 'Miss Efficient' with her clipboard who's there to make the lives of patients and clinicians more difficult. The way managers are portrayed in the mainstream is very unfair and, I believe, damaging. The NHS manager is very 'transactional' in style, as in 'traditional managers making hundreds of transactions every day'. I'm trying to develop people to move beyond that and into leadership. To make transformational change, you need someone to be in leadership mode, which requires them to be much more creative and much more strategic in their intent and analysis. As a psychologist, educationalist and sociologist, I prepare leaders to work in significantly different ways by challenging them about what their value sets and behaviours are, and constantly looking at the tension between the two.

"For example, somebody may think they are very pro-equality, but they may end up appointing a team that is very much in their mould. This is very common, but it is not conscious. Human beings are very comfortable with people who look and sound like them, and who have the same cultural references that they have. In other words, people who think in the same way as they do. The transformational leader is someone who is open to looking at changing himself or herself so they can change services. I would consider it a lifelong task to bring buried values to consciousness. Programmes that just look at behaviours and skills are aimed only at the transactional end. But if you are trying to create really dramatic transformational change, you need people to think creatively.

"But somebody has to be open to that. They have to be up for change in their being as well as their doing. It is what I call 'experiential learning'. I work with emotions in the here and now and how they link to performance. Just tapping into the left linear, logical hemisphere of the brain is not enough. We must use the creative, associative, imaginative, symbolic side of the brain. When you want to bring about real change, the process often begins in a non-traditional or highly creative way."

For example, Valerie takes participants to the National Gallery in London. Now you may well ask "What on earth does art have to do with management in the NHS?" Well, it is the beginning of teaching them about multiple perspectives, to surprise them out of their conventional way of thinking. They work with an art educator and look at only three paintings. With no expert knowledge, they are then asked to create a joint description of what they have learned using shared group knowledge. When they do, they come to realise that collaborating enables good decision-making. It is the same process that makes a difference in a difficult meeting. It begins to open up the whole process of tolerating different viewpoints; partly because they may not know the answer about the paintings because actually there is no right answer. Uncertainty allows ideas and shared learning to flourish."

So how does this translate in a practical way to the real world and some of the more complex problems and challenges faced by managers in today's NHS? Valerie continues: "I think a great part of it is how to listen in a different way. So as a finance director, for example, I might have a commissioner who is very angry about changes in a contract, but by opening up my mind and heart, I can begin to have a dialogue, ride through the anger and get to the core of the problem. Only then can I begin to unravel the real issues and move forward."

A further key set of skills are those that allow a leader to begin to embody leadership, literally for it to imbue their physicality. Valerie explains: "Research shows that only 7% of your impact comes from your words. 37% comes from your intonation, and the remainder from your body language. A good leader has congruence of all of these. We are trying to get people to physically embody the leadership qualities of openness, warmth and collaboration. A leader must put other people at their ease at all times. So we teach people to have learning conversations where they are always searching for new ways of doing things and new approaches to take."

The profile of Valerie and her co-director on the programme, Eden Charles, represent some of these real life challenges. Eden is black, born in St Lucia; Valerie is white, born in a Scottish community in America. They embody the male, the female, the black, the white. Part of the programme is a session where they talk with each other in front of the group for 15 minutes about a topic that interests and engages them both and builds their common ground. Then they will deconstruct the dialogue to trace what went on and understand why; for example, Valerie interrupted Eden at a certain point. Eden and Valerie demonstrate how to use their differences creatively. "We have a conversation and make learning come out of it." Everyone on the programme does the same, both as a speaker and an observer.

Valerie: "It becomes like a board meeting, where you can't have all the air space, yet you need to make sure your interventions are memorable, compelling and make an impact. As a result, participants begin to understand a bit more about their political intelligence. Eden talks about Bi-cultural Competence. The exuberant Jamaican or Mancunian, for instance, has to understand that in board meetings they need to function in a way that is politically effective, yet still stay true to their own cultural roots when in their own cultural milieu. It's like being able to speak fluent French in order to run a business in France when one is British."

Registrars also need to learn a second 'language' when they are making the transition from specialist registrar to consultant. They already have plenty of organising skills, which the programme builds on, while helping them develop the skills and awareness they will need to take on new leadership responsibilities with confidence and authority. The programme also equips them with a thorough understanding of the issues and dynamics that continue to shape the NHS, now and in the future.

In the last two years, Valerie has worked with over 300 specialist registrars (SpRs) who are about to step up to the challenging role of consultant. The programme starts with participants being asked to express frankly their beliefs and feelings about managers; and in many cases they confuse the two. The SpRs learn how to separate their emotional responses from their opinions. Common misconceptions are that managers are 'powerful', 'don't care about patients', are 'career-driven', 'can't get proper jobs' and 'would never survive in industry'. "But we don't judge SpRs for these responses," explains Valerie. "We enable them to work through their prejudices and find creative common ground."

Participants begin to understand the utter complexity of resource decision-making in the NHS, and how, unless they gain this understanding, they end up fighting only for their speciality, which means robbing Peter to pay Paul. "They learn that it is not about cardiology or neurology versus pathology," Valerie notes. "They also learn to appreciate that the manager is trying to hold the equality of resources for patient populations across the whole organisational process. Managers have to look right across the system. And when the registrars see that, they understand managers in a different way. These registrars are very bright people, the crème de la crème of modern medicine. We are not trying to insult them by 'fixing their deficient knowledge base'. We are trying to give them a different perspective. I hope they feel deeply respected yet heavily challenged.

"For their consultant interviews, I teach them how to create an evidence-based answer and how to phrase their achievements in the positive, which is often completely new to them. We emphasise the key importance of their clinical input to whole system collaboration across the manager-clinician divide.

"We then teach them how to ask open-ended questions. For the psychiatrists among them, this is familiar ground, but some of the registrars from other disciplines never do it. They 'tell' people. They don't 'ask'."

The programme raises awareness of the interface between clinical practice and management, and broadens understanding of the role of consultants at corporate level. Participants are encouraged to take responsibility for their own development; they have to explore their own behaviour and capabilities, sharing their experiences and insights with others through group tasks and co-coaching. Ultimately, the objectives are to improve communication skills, recognise the importance of effective team working, gain fresh insights into how systems work, and leave with a network of colleagues from a range of specialisms who can provide ongoing support in the future.

Another important aspect of the programme is the hospital visits that Valerie sets up, the aim of which is to undertake a thorough analysis of the anatomy of the organisation before reporting back. "We say this is a piece of anthropology. An anthropologist will go into another culture, suspend judgment, but be very clear about the prejudices they bring. We challenge the registrars' prejudices about

NHS managers; they have to create an interview schedule of open-ended questions that allows them to test these hypotheses. We do not want a critique of how bad the organisation/managers are, which is what many would like to fall back on. It's their default position.

"You see the artefacts of an organisation the moment you walk in the door – what has it got in the reception area, pots or art? Then you get the mission statement, which enables you to partly understand its culture, then under that you get the unspoken rules, and in the mud you get the roots of what makes the organisation tick. When they do their presentations, we ask them 'What would your life be like if there were no managers?' And they say, 'There would be no strategy, and we would have to run all the systems ourselves.' Without effective leadership, the health service would just not be able to function. It's as simple as that."

Inside-out

THE NHS MAKES a difference. We all know that. But what happens when senior managers move on? Is their training wasted? No. They continue to make a difference, going on to empower other organisations striving to help people in a variety of capacities. This is the story of two managers who have made a real and lasting positive impact, beyond the walls of the NHS, after moving into new positions outside the organisation, using their skills and insights to promote wellbeing in the wider world. The paths of two exceptional women, Barbara Stocking and Olivia Amartey, demonstrate the quality of their NHS training, its strength in new contexts, and their unwavering commitment to being individual forces for good.

BARBARA STOCKING

Barbara Stocking has made as much a name for herself in the charity sector as in her previous incarnation as an NHS regional director and then director of the NHS Modernisation Agency. Since 2001 she has been a director of Oxfam, leading its responses to humanitarian crises in Afghanistan, Iraq and Sudan, and disasters like the tsunami and the Pakistan earthquake. She has strengthened Oxfam's campaigning on issues such as Make Trade Fair, and education, and empowered its development work on livelihoods, HIV/ Aids and climate change. In 2008, her dedication was recognised when she was awarded a DBE. The lessons she absorbed as someone who trained NHS management externally, and then worked internally within the organisation at the highest level, have helped her to steer Oxfam, and its global campaigns for good, safely forward.

Clearly Barbara Stocking has made an extraordinary impact with her life. "I had a very funny sort of training because I didn't actually join the NHS until 1993, so I came in as a regional general manager." Coming in at a very senior position is obviously not the typical entry point. Having worked with the World Health Organisation, Barbara arrived in the NHS via the King's Fund College, "Where I ran the top management programme and most of my formal management training came from going through that programme about four or five times. I was the co-ordinator of the whole thing, but I got any formal training I have had by being a part of that. The rest was done by being in the jobs I have done which have had very strong management content from the beginning."

In terms of her disposition, Barbara admits to being naturally managerial. "I like organising people! That was something in me. When you see a lot of people really working well together and getting somewhere – I just find that enormously satisfying. I was once a staff officer to a very high-level committee in the US looking at the veterans' administration hospital system and even there, just organising a high-level committee in their work and making sure this group worked together well to get to an outcome, I really enjoyed it."

Her background brought Barbara into the orbit of the NHS. "I was at the King's Fund College from 1983, when it was the management training centre for the NHS, fundamentally. It was going through the range of management issues – how you deal with strategic issues, how you design and deliver organisations, how you manage finance, and the whole thing of who you are and managing your own time and yourself. It was a team effort, I co-ordinated it and made it all work, but it was all those other people doing their part. I think people got a lot of different things out of it. Some were at a very high level and they probably just enjoyed the time out and the stimulus of new things and new ideas. A lot of people went on to make life or career changes. Fascinating that you see some people coming on the programme and you find they have gone off in quite different directions. This must be the moment that they know they are ready to move on in their lives. So we had complete changes in and out of the NHS – divorces, babies. These people had come to sort their lives out quite often!"

Crossing the bridge from training people for the NHS to helping to run it directly was a natural progression. "I moved over to be the director of the King's Fund Centre, which was a health service and health and social care development agency, and managed that. It was my first top job. And that was when I first recognised that getting the 150 people working for me really motivated and going, was fantastic. I was working for the health service from the outside, and I just thought, 'I want to be in there doing it, not just doing bits outside,' so I became NHS regional general manager for the Oxford region."

Public service is clearly written through Barbara Stocking like 'Brighton' through a stick of seaside rock. What made her life take that course? "I think it goes back to growing up. My parents were ordinary working class people, my mother stayed at home and my father was a postman in Rugby. They were very much community-oriented people. They were always looking after, worrying about and involved with other people, partly through the Methodist church, where they were very involved. They really believed that everybody had to help each other. This is a tough life; we all need to help each other. But they were part of a community that felt that as well.

"I got to the NHS because I was studying science at university and it went well with healthcare. I came from the sort of background where nobody suggested to me becoming a doctor: that was too grand. From about 18 to about 26 or so, I really kept thinking, 'Should I change over and be a doctor?' And it was only later that I thought, 'Well I am doing some rather interesting things and I'm not sure that I actually do want to be a doctor. I certainly don't want to spend at least five years before I can get near doing anything real.'

"Healthcare was to do with the things I knew about. I had done the work in the US and the WHO work in West Africa. I had done biochemistry and physiology so I felt I knew the subject. The public service aspect I think was absolutely built into me since childhood. And then I think I just really liked the people. The people in the health service are so committed to what they do. Certainly the front line. But even at the managerial level, most people are there because they really want to try to make things better. Maybe also being a woman plays its role. You see quite easily how ill health and health conditions do affect people and how frightening, how difficult it can be, and how people can get really devastated by the way they are treated as well. Certainly by the time I was a regional manager, I felt that very strongly – that how patients get treated really matters. And I led the patient partnership initiative for all the years I was regional director. I felt a real drive for that – how horrible it can be if things go badly, in the sense that, for example, the way someone talks to you at a very critical moment in your life is significant. And how we could make all that better."

Barbara's experiences of the NHS brought enormous and evolving levels of responsibility. "I started in Oxford with four counties to look after. That was in July. In November, Virginia Bottomley said she was going to merge all these regional health authorities into NHS regions. So I got Anglia and Oxford at that point, covering Oxford to Great Yarmouth. I then became regional director for the south east, which was even bigger. South east was eight million people to cover, and the budget was £5 billion.

"When I first got Anglia and Oxford it was the end of the Conservative era and we had rather a good time of it, in that there was freedom, because the Conservatives were not going to do any new health policy. On top of that, as a regional health team, we were really ready to move the region on in terms of healthcare in a really positive way. When I got the south east it was much, much harder. It was just so much bigger. Actually a lot of Sussex, Surrey and Kent had not been managed very thoroughly before, because it had previously been part of London, so all the attention had gone on to the London teaching hospitals because there were so many big issues there. Anyone who was managing that patch was always going to be at the London end rather than out in the counties, and it was very under-managed as a result. Just trying to keep on top of all the things that needed sorting out was a challenge, I don't think I moved that region on in anywhere like the same way as I had done Anglia and Oxford."

In Anglia and Oxford, Barbara views her particular successes as addressing neonatal intensive care, the role of acute hospitals and community hospitals, and trying to build the patient partnership. Her experiences as a manager and a person meant that, "I probably got a lot tougher. Just having to get on and make decisions even if they are quite difficult and difficult for other people really. I always knew that sometimes you do have to move people on from a particular job. It's not very nice but you always know you have to do it. I think the biggest difficulty is always working out whether your judgment is good enough.

"It's about huge juggling: is your judgment right on this one, given that you have got to move so fast? Are you moving too fast, taking the right decisions? We had a lot of capital programmes going on. It was all part of the PFI schemes. Were you really on top of it? That was always the biggest worry. And then were you pushing people too hard? At that time I had very good teams of people. Huge team support. We really worked on things together. People were so experienced. I never had to think 'do they see the problem?' We had complete fluency between us. The support from people there for what I had to do was important because being the boss is lonely. And also they were just good fun. When I was in the NHS I remember having retreats with my regional team where we would get the giggles. It was just a good release."

Moving to Oxfam posed a series of new challenges. "I estimated that when I was regional director for the south east I had 180,000 people working in the health service (for me). If you take the budget and the fact that it was the eighth biggest in England, it was huge, huge, huge. Oxfam is global but the teams are all quite small. The biggest team we had was 700 in Aceh (Indonesia, after the tsunami). So it is a different order of things but then much more complex, because it is in 70 different countries. It is a lot of different businesses, if you like. We also have to make money unlike the NHS. So we are partly a retail trader. We have to do the fundraising

"The real job is alleviating the poverty and suffering. Then within that you have the humanitarian work, which is more like service delivery because we are probably the world's biggest water and sanitation emergency agency. Then you have the campaigning as with Make Poverty History. It's a huge variety. I am always doing something completely different. That's what makes it so exciting. I had 75 chief executives with me in the south east region. Whereas here I have a governance board of 12 people who are absolutely excellent, and who do exert their proper oversight, but who expect me to lead. So as far as I am concerned I can lead and quite quickly take the organisation where it has to go. It's just so liberating.

"The thing I was amused about when I came here was when I was in health there were moments when ministers treated senior managers as a rather lowly breed. And yet most managers were, like me, hugely experienced in healthcare; and really moving in the direction they wanted, oddly enough. When I first came out of the

NHS I would have lunch with Clare Short (when she was Development Secretary) and she treated me like an equal; yet I had just come out of the NHS and I hardly knew anything about development. The difference is clearly I am not accountable to them and Oxfam is very influential. I think all that time in the NHS helped me to understand government and ministers and how to deal with them and what their issues were. In the NHS you really do know how much they have to worry about – the public being concerned about waiting lists and so on. Even though it is making your job more difficult, you understand why they are pressing. I understand the parameters and know what ministers are thinking."

Barbara's successes with Oxfam have been considerable. She cites, "Pushing Tony Blair into doing the Make Poverty History issue; I mean not just me, the whole organisation," as a good example. But ultimately she recognises that, "You don't change big things. You just keep nudging along different bits of it really. We have got an arms' trade treaty going through the UN, which Oxfam and Amnesty have been big backers for. The British government is very supportive of that now. I think they were only lukewarm at first but now they are very keen. And we are keeping them at it. Politicians are always concerned about whether the public are with them. One of our big jobs is to show politicians that there is a public demand. You have to do that in a way that is really snappy and interesting and make them notice and make the media take notice. Then you come to the meetings and negotiation part. I have talked to David Miliband about the arms' trade treaty several times and that is one of many things I talk to him about, and Douglas Alexander as well (Secretary for International Development)."

Culturally, Barbara traces similarities between the NHS and Oxfam. "All the passion you want that drives people is in the organisations, but using your head as well. People wouldn't be here at Oxfam unless they felt moral outrage at what is happening in certain countries. Bringing together the passion and the logic about what to do is quite complicated really. And then you are where the buck stops. Oxfam has been through this for generations. It is 65 years old. A central part of my job is to ensure that Oxfam's reputation and authority is maintained. Very key. I am very happy to be brave, as long as we have really got the facts right and thought it through very carefully. I only get nervous when something comes along and I think we didn't get that quite right."

This has echoes of some of her experiences within the NHS. "I think back to some of the reviews we did, things like Eastbourne hospital where there was very poor management. There it was much more taking it on the chin, really facing up to what had happened. There was some poor management and that led to some very poor nursing. It came out quite starkly in one particular case where a woman died and her family just wanted to make sure that wasn't going to go on. I got the regional nursing director to run an investigation. And it was pretty bad. I am very proud that we brought it right out into the open and then dealt with the problem. There was no hiding about that; it was the NHS straightforwardly saying 'there is a big hospital failing people here'. It was right trying to push the NHS to be much more accountable and transparent. Which I really believed in."

Belief. Perhaps that has been the key to Barbara Stocking's career success as a woman who has made such a difference with her management skills.

OLIVIA AMARTEY

Olivia Amartey was a graduate of the NHS Management Training Scheme and has worked in various management roles within the NHS and beyond. She then made a life-changing decision to take a job with the Church of England as director of social responsibility with the Diocese of Lichfield. Her role was to promote participation with the diocese and to work with agencies to make sure issues of justice and care were being addressed. She also founded her own charity, Martha's Oasis and created the Sisters with Voices Personal Development Programme, for young teen women. This charity, after being featured in Channel 4's 'The Secret Millionaire', secured a sizeable donation from the secret millionaire participant. Coming full circle, Olivia returned with her skills back to the NHS in Birmingham's inner city, which incorporates the Perry Barr area where she was born. Clearly her journey has enabled her to apply her training and skills in numerous capacities to benefit society.

Olivia was born in Birmingham to a Jamaican family where the ethos was to work hard and get ahead. She became a radiographer in the NHS. "I wanted to combine science with serving people and became a diagnostic radiographer. I especially enjoyed trauma radiography. For example, a patient would come in with an injury such as a broken bone, or severe pain and you had to bring all your skills to bear to operate the complex X-ray machinery and position the patient to get the views needed by the doctors and surgeons. You are an integral part of the A&E and emergency care team. I saw my work and myself as a crucial link in the chain, making an impact on the patient pathway to gain the best possible outcome for them."

Her ambition led Olivia to search for a way of progressing in the NHS. "I was in my mid 20s and had worked my way up to become a senior radiographer. However, promotion above a certain grade was, at that time, very difficult and I was ambitious. I looked at the superintendent radiographers and I thought 'I want to move on, run the department'. I remember thinking, 'Why do I have to wait for someone to die or retire to get where I want to be?' I went for a job as superintendent radiographer at a children's hospital with several years of radiography under my belt. I was turned down flat because I hadn't progressed through all the proper grades and levels. It made me really mad because I knew I could do the job. So I started to explore management as a career option and I decided to upgrade my radiographer diploma to a degree by embarking on a fast-track course. This meant travelling to Edinburgh every other weekend.

My applications to junior management positions within the hospital failed. It was at this point that I came across the NHS Management Training Scheme by typing 'NHS management' into Google. I went and spoke to someone in HR who was a graduate of the scheme itself. She told me it was extremely competitive, but an excellent scheme. I applied, was shortlisted and went onto the 24-hour assessment and selection centre."

Olivia was one of 60 chosen from 2,000 applicants nationwide. During the assessment process she was unsure of her performance. "I am the one who sits back and observes everyone else. I thought I am not contributing to this exercise, but I was watching how everyone else in the group was interacting with each other and in the process completely discarding crucial pieces of information. At key moments I would say, 'But you have missed this and have you thought about the impact of that decision?' With hindsight I was acting in a strategic overview role. I didn't know this was in me, but I recognise that's the way I work. I'm not in the scrum. I seem to operate best by keeping at a distance, but it is a very helpful distance. Later I was told that one of the reasons I was selected was because of my lightning fast answer to what I thought was a very patronising question asked by the interviewer. It involved going into a supermarket and buying washing powder and working out a mathematical calculation. I answered: 'What sort of question is that – do you think I am stupid?' Afterwards, one of the assessors told me they realised I was the sort of person they were looking for – someone who had guts enough to challenge things they thought were wrong."

Joining the programme had a deep effect on Olivia. "As well as gaining managerial skills, we would hear from chief executives of hospital trusts and engage in debate and discussions with people from health-related think-tanks such as the King's Fund. We were also thinking big ideas about how health managers could make significant and positive differences, in practice, to patients. So we asked the really big questions, such as 'Will healthcare continue to be free or is it inevitable that we will migrate to an insurance-based system?' My rationale was to use this training opportunity to my best advantage. My mentor was the chief executive of the Princess Royal hospital, Telford; his enthusiasm was so inspiring. I just thought: 'This is so exciting – we can change this, we can change the way healthcare is delivered.'

"We were assigned as trainee managers to a particular hospital through a matching process. I ended up working in Oswestry on the Welsh border. I had to drive 150 miles there and back every day but I loved it there. It was a small orthopaedic hospital with a national reputation for sports injuries. I was assigned as the operational manager in charge of day surgery, physiotherapy and occupational therapy and the day hospital. My role was essentially to manage the day-to day issues, review the existing services and make improvements. As a small hospital with relatively few senior managers and a flat hierarchy, it meant I was a big fish in a small pond and therefore exposed to a lot of strategic decisions and decision-making processes.

"I was directly involved with the executive team and given large-scale projects to complete. One project was to review the role of the REACT (rapid emergency assessment team) and explore how their work could improve the day hospital services. Another big piece of work involved reviewing the contracts of one specialist area of orthopaedics, where cartilage was grown for use in knee replacement surgery. As a then cutting edge piece of research, my task was to explore the cost-effectiveness of keeping this work 'in-house' or commissioning it to an outside specialist company. I recommended that the hospital should hold onto its intellectual property and continue to develop the service. I reasoned that although it would lose money in the short term, its development would gain the Trust kudos, and 'world leader' status. So it was taking a long-term view over the short term. They accepted my recommendation.

"The three-month elective element of the training scheme

allowed us to choose, work and study a particular aspect of health-care and this could be undertaken either in the UK or abroad. The objective was to bring back this key learning to the NHS. I chose to go Atlanta, Georgia, in the United States to work as a project manager at The Office of Minority Health. Its mission was to make health services accessible to blacks, Hispanics, Asians and other ethnicities that had difficulty with mainstream services. My aims were to find out what healthcare was like in a society where there were massive divisions, along economic and racial lines. However, I soon found out that I couldn't affect any change or progress my projects because of the internal politics that I was blissfully unaware of. The job was desk-based and I soon grew bored with its imposed limitations. After a chance meeting with the friend of a colleague, I changed my job midway through my elective. I went to work as project assistant with The United Way – a USA-wide organisation who wanted a strategic person to co-ordinate their philanthropic projects with huge multi-national corporations like Atlanta Bell and Coca-Cola."

Olivia had acquired an invaluable skills base, having worked in a clinical environment and with her trainee experience in management and liaison with various external organisations. Unsurprisingly, upon graduation, she found herself in demand. "I was headhunted to take a position at the George Eliot hospital in Nuneaton, to lead the patient and public involvement agenda and develop training courses for the hospital's staff and clinicians. This involved empowering patients with the necessary skills to engage with clinicians, sit on the hospital's patient forum and take part in nurse training courses. I was later promoted to assistant, then general manager of surgery and orthopaedics. In this role I had to work closely with clinicians to manage services as well as the budget and the staff that came with it. The job involved a whole gamut of things. You have to work with a wide range of other departments – for example diagnostics and theatres, as their efficient working is critical to the success of your own service. I helped restructure day surgery to improve care for our patients."

After that Olivia went to University Hospitals Birmingham as group manager for medicine and respiratory medicine. She developed strong project management skills there, working under the managerial leadership of Mark Britnell, then chief executive of the Trust. "His leadership style was charismatic and dynamic. His remarkable memory meant that you could never be complacent around him. Out of nowhere he would ask your opinion on a project or aspect of your service that you were developing. This served to keep us on our toes."

In 2006 Olivia left the NHS in search of new challenges. "An opportunity came up out of the blue. In the Church of England they wanted to have a fresh look at social action. I applied for the job as director of social responsibility and was the only non-cleric selected. At interview I spoke passionately about the similarities between the NHS and the Church and how both of these organisations exist to make a permanent and significant difference in the lives of its users. My managerial experiences prepared me well to look critically at a service and identify how we could make things better, relevant and accessible."

Having won the job, Olivia was faced with the challenge of applying her experience and strategic skills in her new environment. "I was working for the Bishop of Lichfield looking at how the Church can be a significant factor in people's lives. Not only in terms of the religious experience, but how the social responsibility arm of the Church can be used to good effect, to serve ordinary people in real and relevant ways. I wanted to make the Church accessible not only in word but in deed. I started by looking at what already existed as a vehicle for social change and how we could change or magnify its effects to make it relevant to people – not only Church members but also those who never set foot there. What I discovered was that there is a great energy in the Church for making a difference. Many

Church members are extremely motivated and want to reach out and engage with the often messy and real stuff of people's lives and so set up projects or initiatives to address the identified gaps apparent in their communities. On another, more strategic level, we looked at which organisations the diocese needed to partner with.

"I set about mapping and cataloguing the projects the Church was already doing in the diocese – for example, those working with the police, youth offending teams, prisons, older persons, young children and families in crisis. One key piece of research was undertaken jointly with the Saltbox, an intermediary agency based in Stoke-on-Trent. Together we produced a comprehensive Staffordshire-wide report that detailed the excellent work that all faith groups contributed to the aims and objectives of the Local Area Agreement. For example, we said to the county services, 'You want to do something about homeless people, but did you know there is (a church) group here that feeds 50 homeless people, picking up the pieces of their lives and signposting them on, and your official figures say there are only four homeless people in the county?' In monetary terms, the Church was saving Staffordshire County Council over a million pounds per year. It was the first time that the work of faith groups was assigned a monetary value. This had a great impact on the county's statutory agencies and highlighted the value of voluntary work.

"Faith groups don't want to change their ethos. They remain on the frontline long after statutory agencies have moved on to focus on other priorities. The challenge is to break down the barriers with which one views the other. Statutory groups believe the Church is only involved in social action because it wants to convert everyone. And faith groups are wary of being target driven. So they were suspicious of each other. I drew on my experience as an NHS manager to challenge the organisational arrogance that can be displayed by both sides, as each believes that they alone have the answer and know what is best for the client. I identified that if the Church was to become a service provider we needed to sit at the table with health, probation, and statutory housing services as equal partners. Because of the strategic management training I'd had in the NHS, I knew who to go and talk to and I wasn't afraid to do so. By nature clergy are woefully self-deprecating and it was my belief that they needed to sing and dance about the excellent work they were doing."

Olivia's commitment to changing society for the better extended into her personal life and she founded a charity: Martha's Oasis. "It allows women the space to exhale. We reach out to teen girls and women through programmes and services that allow them to make significant life choices." One of Martha's Oasis' programmes is the Sisters With Voices personal development programme aimed at young women aged 13–17. The charity was featured on Channel 4's 'The Secret Millionaire', where an undercover millionaire works with local groups before deciding which one to fund. It won £25,000. After being featured, "We were flooded with enquiries and our website crashed. We have had people from all over the country asking about buying the programme for their organisation. We are now working with Kavita Oberoi (the millionaire) nationally to roll it out across the country."

Olivia has come full circle, now working as a project manager at the Heart of Birmingham Teaching PCT on 'Towards 2010' – a huge programme of change to move healthcare into the heart of the patients' communities. She has contributed so much beyond the NHS and now brings back into the organisation a wealth of new insights and experiences.

A new breed

ONCE THERE WERE three channels on television. A mobile phone was something stuck into the wall with a long flex. A computer filled a room. It's always difficult to see the shape of the future. However, a new breed of manager is entering the NHS with a fresh and distinctive perspective that sees management and medicine as partners, rather than oppositional cultures. Roshelle Ramkisson is a doctor who has just begun her NHS management career by joining the North West Deanery Medical Leadership Programme, having chosen to specialise in psychiatry. Her diverse background and hybrid insights make her very much the shape of things to come.

Roshelle's background spans continents and cultures, being ethnically Indian but raised in South Africa. "As a child I was fortunate to have travelled to various countries around the world and learnt about different ways of life. My last two years of high school, four and a half years of medical school, and one year as a house officer in a hospital, were spent in India, Bangalore. I then returned to South Africa for a period before coming to the UK."

In India, she was required to complete a placement in the government sector called community service as a part of preventive and social medicine. "It was fascinating and also incredibly touching."

Her experiences going out into the villages of India were field medicine at its most raw. "You would have a bag of medications but only a handful of different drugs in there, for example we had two types of antibiotics. In a group of three doctors, we would visit a particular area and screen about 250 children at a time, hoping that we might find something in our medical bag to help. We would try to get more complex cases referred to a local hospital but this was often complicated by the cost as most of the people we saw had very little money. People were really grateful for even the smallest thing you did."

Roshelle then decided to specialise in psychiatry. It is perhaps the perfect background for a manager with its emphasis on insight and dialogue. She left India, and started a clinical attachment in Bedford and Luton Mental Health and Social Care Partnership NHS Trust. "I literally got a crash course in psychiatry. I got much more experience of patients and their problems and just as importantly, having come from another country, got a feel for the system of the NHS, how teams work and so on.

"I started to gain experience in the various specialist teams made up of individuals with a variety of skills. I began to experience, and started to read about, the pros and cons of these teams. I loved it. I absolutely loved it. Understanding people, understanding problems, and I could be in a position to help them, as opposed to figuring out what medications I had in this bag of mine. And from every patient I learn something different, because each of them has their own lives, their own story to tell."

It didn't take long before Roshelle's natural inclination to manage services in the best possible way emerged. "In the early intervention service one of the doctors there got me involved in trying to find comparative data from 60 patients who weren't in the service and 60 who were. The service picks up people who present with a first episode of psychosis and then after three years they discharge them back to the community service. That got me thinking about systems and management. I like the idea of care, free at the point of delivery, but it's got to be the right care. We were looking, through the epidemiology, of what was the best way to manage people, at the end of three years. I became far more aware of the systems in place and how it can have an impact on people. Three of my clinical consultants were doctors with a significant role in management and leadership. I saw the difference they were able to make."

When Roshelle began her specialist training it provided an even greater insight into the impact management can make. "I got a job for Greater Manchester West NHS Foundation Trust doing basic specialist training. Here again I became involved in exploring the effect of a service by auditing the pathway of care in the memory clinics. It was taking months for patients with a diagnosis of dementia to be prescribed anti-dementia drugs. Here were people who really needed help. The trust used that evidence to try to negotiate more funds and resources for the services. Now they have four more community psychiatric nurses, some admin staff, and some scanners and computers. I am about to re-audit the service hoping that the resources will have had a positive effect on the patient pathway."

Roshelle believes that the oppositional stances that can arise between managers and clinicians can be solved by remembering that both are serving patients' interests, and looking to two main areas: "Communication and engaging people. I think the medical director of the Trust here treads a nice line between the clinicians and the managers. I have been very impressed with that. He always tries to look at the patient experience and patient care. That means a lot to me. It goes back to my experiences of patients who didn't have very much, and yet who were so grateful for what you could do for them."

It is perhaps this enjoyment of listening to people and connecting with them to improve things, together with her commitment to making a tangible difference that led Roshelle into the North West Deanery Medical Leadership Programme. She has now embarked on a journey that will ultimately see her joining the ranks of senior managers. The programme has been designed to develop doctors with the potential to fast track into senior leadership positions. Its eight trainees work closely with those on the NHS North West Graduate Management Training Scheme in an attempt to create positive working relations between doctors and managers at the outset of their careers as leaders. The programme directors were looking for people with exceptional motivation to take on the responsibilities of leadership. Roshelle had already demonstrated it. "The programme itself is challenging yet exciting. We have been given immense support from the deanery and it is indeed a wonderful opportunity. We have hands on vocational management exposure, an academic component and our clinical training, which would not be possible to achieve without the efforts of an associate dean, support manager, programme directors, consultants and professors to name a few."

There can sometimes be a sense of 'them and us' between clinicians and managers, but Roshelle, with a foot in both camps, has a clear viewpoint on this. "Some people fear or despise managers. We have to, as part of our diploma work, make appointments with managers/leaders and find out about their styles, what influences them. I am gaining an understanding of where they are coming from and about the environment they work in as well as the attitudes of the people in an organisation. I don't see them as being as 'evil' as other people would make them out to be. I am learning to stand back and visualise the bigger picture. The irony of the perceived differences is that both clinicians and managers want the same thing – improvement of patient care." She sees the biggest battle between the two NHS cultures as frequently arising from, "little misunderstandings that can harden over time, when you get set in your ways."

"Most of us have been, or know a loved one who has been, a patient at some point and I am no exception. I know what it is like to be on the receiving end in hospital, or having a test, or waiting for your medication. It makes you think about smoothing the system, planning and so on. Alongside the impact of powerful medications and life saving procedures, we should not forget all the people vital to the process of recovery, for example the lady serving dinner that makes the extra effort to smile warmly and find something for all the patients, encouraging them to eat so that they regain their strength sooner.

"I have to say that even though we get caught up in the politics of it, you do get a sense in the NHS that people care. Communication is one of the key ingredients in the recipe for improvement, as well as a large dollop of patience for our patients. By that I mean that even with the fast pace of life in the twenty-first century, where time is money, we need to slow down in the business of health. The NHS is a system run by people for people. To be most effective, we need to be patient with one another as providers of care, as well with those we are here to serve."

View from the top

SIR RICHARD BRANSON. Damien Hirst. Bono. Rupert Murdoch. Peter Jones. Willie Walsh. David Nicholson. Sir Timothy Leahy. Jonathan Ross. Sir Alex Ferguson. Delia Smith. Lewis Hamilton. Theo Paphitis. Simon Cowell. Sir Alan Sugar. Philip Green. Richard and Judy. Sir Terence Conran. Kate Moss. David Beckham. JK Rowling. Chris Martin.

If the UK general public was asked to list the aforementioned in terms of how influential they are, it is highly probable that David Nicholson would come somewhere near the bottom of that list. But forget about sports, holidays, music, media, fashion, football, motor racing, wizardry, gossip or fine dining, because David Nicholson is ultimately responsible for a service that most people cherish above all else: the National Health Service. As its chief executive, it is often said that David heads the world's third largest organisation after the Indian railways and Wal-Mart. It makes Philip Green's high street fashion empire look more like a corner shop.

VIEW OF THE CHIEF EXECUTIVE

"The Next Stage Review (NSR) is our plan and vision for the NHS over the next 10 years. Our ambition is to significantly improve services for patients, using quality as our organising principle. Led by eminent surgeon, Professor Lord Ara Darzi, the Review involved 60,000 NHS staff, 2,000 clinicians and stakeholders and partner agencies; a level of involvement and engagement unprecedented in the history of the service.

"The NHS is now moving to the implementation phase. The local NHS, stakeholders and partner agencies are working together – supported by the Department of Health – to take their plans forward. No one underestimates the challenge of this scale of change in the largest integrated public health system in the world.

"We have looked across the globe for evidence about large scale change – what works and what doesn't. The evidence shows that leadership which is absolutely focused on the customer, on the patient, on the community, makes a bigger difference than one that is focused on the bureaucracy and the centre. I call this looking out, not up. Not leaders who patrol the boundaries of their organisations. We need leaders who look out, to patients, communities, partner agencies; leaders who understand the needs and aspirations of their local communities. That may seem obvious, but we traditionally have had real difficulty in taking that forward.

"The government will always have a view, given that it funds the NHS to the tune of over £100 billion pounds a year. That's obvious, but we need to change the nature and quality of the leadership that we exhibit. We can learn, we can develop, we need to think about our own experiences, we need to think about the way in which we ourselves interact with the service. This relentless focus on our patients and on our communities is absolutely essential to get the kind of leadership to take the service through this big change."

David Nicholson,
NHS Chief Executive
Extract from speech to East Midlands NHS event
October 2008

Working with the NHS Management Board, which includes 10 director generals, David's appointment in September 2006 has already brought about some significant changes: services have improved, patient waiting times have been cut considerably, and the financial position of the organisation has been transformed from a deficit to half a billion pounds surplus. The future has already begun.